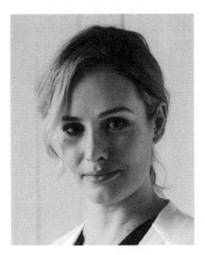

Dr Nikki Stamp FRACS is a cardiothoracic surgeon,
one of only 11 female heart surgeons in Australia.
Her clinical work is at the forefront of cardiothoracic surgery,
including transplants and congenital heart disease.
She has a particular interest in women's heart disease and how
the medical system can better serve female patients.
Nikki has hosted heart health episodes for Australia's flagship
science TV programme, *Catalyst,* as well as *Operation Live,*
in which she commentated a live caesarean birth.
Her first book, *Can You Die of a Broken Heart?,*
has been translated into seven languages.

Published in 2019 by Murdoch Books,
an imprint of Allen & Unwin

Copyright © Nikki Stamp 2019

Murdoch Books Australia
83 Alexander Street, Crows Nest NSW 2065
Phone: +61 (0)2 8425 0100
murdochbooks.com.au
info@murdochbooks.com.au

Murdoch Books UK
Ormond House, 26–27 Boswell Street, London WC1N 3JZ
Phone: +44 (0) 20 8785 5995
murdochbooks.co.uk
info@murdochbooks.co.uk

A catalogue record for this book is available from the National Library of Australia

A catalogue record for this book is available from the British Library
ISBN 978 1 76052 454 8 Australia
ISBN 978 1 91163 234 4 UK

Cover design by Alissa Dinallo
Author photograph by Chris Chen
Printed and bound in Australia by Griffin Press

10 9 8 7 6 5 4 3 2 1

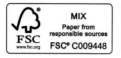

DR NIKKI STAMP

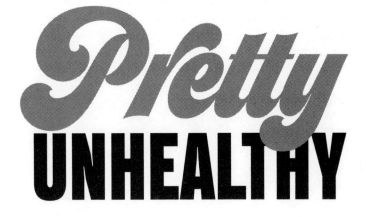

Pretty UNHEALTHY

Why our obsession with looking healthy is making us sick

murdoch books
Sydney | London

CONTENTS

✦ ✦ ✦

INTRODUCTION:
WAKE-UP CALL

✚ ✚ ✚

The cuff tightened on my left arm. I could tell by how tight it was getting that the result was not going to be good. When it finally released, I looked at the numbers on the screen.

Shit. My blood pressure was way too high.

My doctor looked over his glasses and raised his eyebrows. He pressed the button again, hopefully to show us both that there was nothing wrong and that this ridiculously high blood pressure was just a mistake; a one-off.

After months and months of feeling so tired that I struggled to make it through most days, I had finally gone to see my doctor. For a long time, I had put it down to working too hard and burning the candle at both ends. I had finally reached a point where I couldn't stand the fatigue that I could feel in my bones; I decided to stop being a doctor who was dismissing all her symptoms and go and be a patient.

For the second time, the cuff around my arm released and made an audible sigh. And for the second time, the number was too high.

'I can't really accuse you of having white coat hypertension, can I?' he said, referring to the artificially high blood pressure people get when confronted with a doctor. I think we both assumed

I would be immune to that, as a doctor myself. All I could do was give him a nervous laugh as he pressed the button again, hoping for third time lucky.

There was no such luck, and the numbers on the screen stared back at me accusingly. We decided that after months of high blood pressure – something that runs in my family – it was time for some treatment. I also had to have a battery of blood tests to check for other reasons why I might be so tired. I left his office clutching a prescription for a blood pressure medication; I also bought a home blood pressure monitor to check myself. I was, on the inside at least, a little ashamed and a little scared.

Just a few days after starting my tablets, I felt amazing. My blood pressure was much lower and I had so much energy. Rather than waking up every morning feeling like I hadn't slept at all for months, when my alarm went off I was bright and ready to face the day. I couldn't remember the last time I had felt so good. So healthy.

Outwardly, I blamed my newfound diagnosis squarely on my genetics. When my friends and colleagues marvelled that I was too young and looked far too healthy to have high blood pressure, let alone be on treatment for it, I blamed my dad. He has been treated for high blood pressure since his 20s. I laughed and said something along the lines of: 'You can't choose your parents.'

Inwardly, I knew that this wasn't entirely fair. I knew that even with the genetic make-up for things like high blood pressure or heart disease, living a healthy lifestyle slashes your risk of actually developing the illness. I knew that I had really not been taking care of myself, letting my exercise lapse and eating foods that were easy and fast, but almost certainly not that healthy. I knew I was over-committed and over-stressed. But I had managed to hide these feelings and pretend that everything was fine. After all, I *looked* fine. It was an easy lie to get away with when the outside appearances hid the inside problems.

About a week after my doctor's visit, I was in a changing room, trying on a dress in one of my favourite stores. I was cursing the fact that the room had no mirror and I needed to venture outside into the public eye to see if I looked any good. I hate doing that; I get self-conscious about what other people will see. I wanted to judge myself, my body and my appearance in private. As I wrestled with the zip at the back of the dress, my phone beeped with a message.

It read: 'Nikki, your fasting blood sugar is a bit high. I have added an HbA1c to check you don't have diabetes. I'm sure it's probably okay though.' An HbA1c is a blood test that gives a picture of how high someone's blood sugars have been over the past six weeks – I know it well because I often order it for my own patients.

I felt the blood drain from my face. My head was filled with doctor thoughts, muddled with fear. *Do I have diabetes? Maybe I don't have diabetes, just pre-diabetes... But, Nikki, that's also bad*, I told myself.

The sales assistant yelled into the changing room: 'Going okay in there?' *No*, I thought, *I might have bloody diabetes*. Surely not though. I looked down at the dress and ventured out to the communal mirror, my brain still going a million miles an hour to decipher what the hell was wrong with me. I stared at my reflection and the thoughts that came next were not good: *I can't get diabetes. I can't be unhealthy; look, I'm not even fat. This dress is a small. People who wear small size dresses can't have diabetes.*

My more realistic (and harsher) brain kicked in: *You know very well that is complete bullshit. Firstly, you are not fat, but that doesn't mean that you can't have diabetes or high blood pressure. Secondly, be honest: you have been taking really bad care of yourself, you're eating badly, you're not exercising and those few extra kilos you've gained, that's why we're here. Small size or not, you're unhealthy.* I felt like I was being told off, which I probably should have been.

The sales assistant must have assumed I was deep in thought over my dress, not weighing up in my head the risk of having a heart attack or mentally going through the exercise I had avoided in the last week. I bought the dress, maybe in an effort to prove that I am small and therefore worthwhile and definitely not sick, and scurried out of the shop.

What had gone so wrong? Not just with my health, but with my thinking? Why was I trying to rationalise my wellbeing with my looks and my size? Why was I so quick to dismiss hard evidence of a problem off the back of the picture I posted on Instagram last week in which I looked pretty good? Why was the label on a dress a more important marker of my health than the fact that I was on medication for blood pressure?

I had been sucked in, that's why. Sucked in by a lifetime of exposure to incorrect information and disordered thinking. I had been told that the way I looked was the most important thing and the most important marker of how healthy I was. I had scrolled through social media and flipped through magazines that sold me messages on how to 'drop that last 5 kilos quick' which backed on to articles about how 'every body was beautiful'. No wonder I was confused: the messages I had received my whole life were bewildering and they were dangerous.

Despite the fact that as a heart surgeon I spend every single day battling illness that has its roots in the way we live our lives, I had let my own health slip. Not only that, I was just as vulnerable to the flawed messages about health equalling beauty. I'd been taking advice from beautiful 20-something women whose Instagram posts showed a life purporting to be healthy, but which were, in fact, heavily filtered and often filled with inaccurate information.

The end product of all of this? It would seem that I was, in fact, pretty unhealthy.

Weighing up the options

Sitting across from me is a young woman. She has an aneurysm of her aorta, the main blood vessel out of the heart, and she needs an operation to fix it. The surgery will probably take me about five hours or more and it's up there with one of the biggest surgeries anyone could ever need. She is otherwise generally well, apart from having high blood pressure. A little like me, she tells me that it 'runs in her family' and she has no idea how she got it.

I feel quite relaxed as I explain to her the problem, why we need to fix it and exactly how I would do that. These are the conversations I have day in and day out; I draw diagrams and the words to tell people what is happening to them roll off my tongue.

This woman, however, has another problem that I do not really want to talk to her about. My comfort is replaced with a low-level anxiety as I start to talk about her weight and her lifestyle. I always ask my patients if they exercise and what their diet is like; this patient tells me that she spends a lot of time on computers and doesn't do any exercise. She is very overweight and, while it is a term that is highly medicalised and not at all pleasant, she meets the criteria for obesity. This has nothing to do with her self-worth or any judgements about her as a person, but is relevant to the impending surgery. It worries me because overweight or obese patients undergoing this surgery have a significantly higher risk of problems, including potentially disastrous wound infections. When you are already facing major surgery, you need all the odds stacked in your favour, not against you.

I take a deep breath and tell her we'll need to be extra vigilant about complications. I can feel her anxiety as I talk: I bet I'm not the first doctor or the last to explicitly or otherwise talk about her weight and lifestyle. I tell her I need her to get fitter for surgery and refer her to an outpatient exercise program where she can learn how to move her body. We're stacking the odds here, I explain. I make referrals to a dietitian and an appointment to see her again before surgery in six weeks' time.

As she leaves, I feel guilty. I think it's because I am so afraid of shaming someone about their body. Our society has equated being fat with a litany of negative things about that person. We stereotype them as unworthy, lazy and unattractive. We inflict immense shame on people because of their outward appearance, and often we do this under the guise of talking about health.

I have a very good reason to talk to people about the way they live their lives. Whether it's about exercising, stopping smoking or improving their diet for the health of their hearts, it is a part of my job and integral to the care I need to give people. And yet, I am quite often scared to have these discussions because the last thing I want people to feel is ashamed of who they are. I also know of patients who have had these discussions with their doctors, and then make complaints to the hospital that someone mentioned their weight or told them they absolutely have to stop smoking.

We have long since stopped thinking of health in terms of what our bodies can do. Rather, we have become conditioned to see health as the superficial behaviours or appearance of someone's body. We judge the health of our own and others' lives by the size of their clothes and the food in their shopping trolley. We live in a world where a picture-perfect healthy lifestyle has become more important to achieve than actual health itself.

We never talk honestly or openly about how healthy we actually are, what our bodies can and can't do. We're not honest with the way we eat, hiding away binges and ultra-restrictive diets in equal measure. We take advice from someone with a social media account or a blog as gospel in our quest to at least appear healthy and follow this advice without ever questioning if it is actually good for us. We never show how bad we feel about our bodies as we scroll through photos of beautiful people, hoping to discover inspiration but finding shame and confusion instead.

Now, I am angry with this state of affairs.

I am furious at the false story we've been sold for years, equating health with how we look, and that we're sold false promises and snake oil by people and industries who bank on us feeling bad about ourselves. When I see a patient, the fact that I am afraid to talk to them about their health for fear of making them feel ashamed is frustrating. Despite my education, my training and my exposure to health and disease, I am still susceptible to the misleading messages of health and wellbeing, and that infuriates me.

As a society, we have lost sight of what it is to be truly healthy: to have bodies that are resilient to disease, and able to do everything we want them to do, and to feel emotionally fulfilled. Instead, we have become obsessed with an ideal: with losing weight fast, fitness fads and superficial judgements about how healthy or unhealthy people appear.

I want to change all of that. I want to take a wrecking ball to these false assumptions and create a new normal, where we look after our bodies for optimal health not just to appear healthy. To do this will mean dismantling decades of beliefs about our bodies and what constitutes health.

It is a long overdue change – for us to finally love our bodies rather than to hate them. To finally think critically about the vast information we are fed and to change our focus from looking good to actually, truly being healthy. I'm excited to embark on this revolution, which will lead to real and all-encompassing health.

Chapter 1

SICK ENOUGH
YET?

'Pick one: gym floor or hospital floor.'

ANONYMOUS

I got home from work late following an emergency surgery. I had been operating on a middle-aged man who had suffered a bigger heart attack than we had thought and it took my team and me hours working well into the night to save his life. As I finally got to bed I promised myself that I would still go for a run in the morning. My body needed it. 'No excuses, just get it done,' I told myself.

Of course, when the alarm sounded at 5:30am, I stared at it through bleary eyes, craned my neck to hear the strong gusts of wind outside and pulled the covers up a little tighter to keep out the cold. When I surfaced, still pretty tired, I told myself off.

On my ward that morning, as every morning, patients displayed the end results of years of lifestyle disease. In one room was a 48-year-old woman who'd had a heart attack and been operated on earlier in the week. Next door was a man in a wheelchair, his leg missing above the knee on one side and the dusky stump on the other side finishing just below the knee. I knew it wouldn't be long before that ended above the knee too. A relative of his walked past me and I could smell the cigarette smoke wafting after them.

The television screen in a patient's room showed yet another health story with an aggressive headline: 'Australians are getting fatter and sicker.' I wondered if a lifetime of late nights leading to missed morning runs was going to put me in the same predicament.

Throughout human history, until fairly recently, infectious diseases have struck us down time and time again. Epidemics of infections such as dysentery, influenza or smallpox have wiped out vast swathes of the population. For instance, the Spanish flu killed an estimated 75 million people in the early twentieth century. Millions have died globally from outbreaks of cholera, dysentery and smallpox. With the advent of better public health including hygiene campaigns, vaccinations and antibiotics, we have largely innoculated ourselves against these kinds of illnesses, especially in developed countries.

Now we face a different threat. Around the world, 70 per cent of deaths result from non-communicable diseases: diseases of our lifestyle, not spread by bacteria or the other enemies of earlier generations, but caused by the way we treat our bodies. The main culprits are heart disease and diabetes caused by smoking, inactivity, poor nutrition, alcohol use and obesity. For the first time in decades, life expectancy in the United States is declining. The threat to the length and quality of our lives has a lot to do with these lifestyle diseases. In affluent countries we have the money and resources to both fuel and battle this modern plague, but it also affects people in developing countries. Nobody is safe from the growing danger.

Even for those of us who are living longer, this is coupled with an enormous burden of disease. More people than ever before have high blood pressure and diabetes, meaning a lifetime of medication, doctors' visits or operations. Heart disease and strokes, of which a staggering 80 per cent are preventable, now cost more lives and more health-care dollars than other medical conditions or injuries such as road trauma. Tobacco consumption still claims more lives around the world, but inactivity, obesity and diet are not far behind. If we get the extra years out of our time here on this planet, they may well be tarnished with disease.

And it's not just heart disease and diabetes. Did you know bowel cancer, breast cancer, throat cancer, stroke, emphysema and even dementia all have proven associations with poor diet, exercise, alcohol use and smoking? Estimates from multiple research studies and the World Health Organization (WHO) state that around a third of cancers could be prevented by a healthy lifestyle. Heart disease risk could be halved, and yet so many of us struggle with this, despite knowing what we should do. For me, the hardest part of this growing epidemic of illness is not the money it costs us: it's the lives and the quality of the days we live that really hurt. These aren't just numbers on a page to me. These are my reality; this is the enemy I wrestle with on a daily basis. Countless times, I have heard patients and doctors alike say, 'If only'. If only I had done more of this or less of that, then I wouldn't be so sick. I wouldn't be having heart surgery as a young man. I wouldn't be staring down a cancer diagnosis. I could do the things that I want.

We're getting sicker earlier in life and we have no idea what to do about it. Or perhaps we do know some of what is good for us, but actually doing those healthy things is really challenging. In our desperation, we turn to pictures of beautiful girls selling 'flat tummy teas' (a 'tea' that is in fact just a laxative or diuretic) as our inspiration for health. We diet ourselves into misery and failure. We run long distances as a form of punishment for eating too much, rather than to nurture ourselves. We have allowed our society to place advertising dollars and false science ahead of real health. And we carry the shame of never being quite good enough.

The O word

Obesity is not a nice word. Just saying it tends to conjure up unflattering images in our minds. But it's a medical term that needs examining. Uncomfortable as it may be, it's time to get real about obesity, overweight and the dreaded F-word – fat. Medically speaking, obesity is defined as having a body mass index (BMI) over 30. BMI is a simple calculation of dividing your weight (in kilograms) by your height (in metres squared). It's got some important limitations as a measure of health but it has a place in this discussion. When you have a BMI over 25, you're classed as overweight. Over 40 and it's called severe obesity.

The more overweight you are, the more likely you are to have health problems. When people refer to obesity as an epidemic, it's a shocking reference to how quickly so many of us have got bigger. The rates of severe obesity in the US quadrupled between 1986 and 2000. More than half the population in developed countries is considered overweight, and in Europe, Australia and the US almost 30 per cent are obese, according to government statistics.

Childhood obesity is a growing problem with a third of American children and adolescents now overweight or obese. In

Australia, the number of overweight children has risen dramatically to the point where one in four kids is now overweight. Those children are more at risk of becoming overweight adults and developing all the associated health problems. Kids who are overweight are also particularly vulnerable to the crippling social stigma that comes with looking that way; this can lead to a lack of focus on encouraging them to be healthy.

It's no secret that our modern lives have contributed to this problem. We're acutely aware of how little physical activity we do and how easy it is to access energy-dense and nutrient-poor foods. We know the effect of poor-quality sleep and how much our phones and computers do for us. We quite literally do not need to get off the couch to carry out our lives.

We used to tell ourselves that obesity came as the result of a fatal character flaw: laziness. I still hear colleagues explaining someone's obesity as the end result of lack of willpower or not wanting to change enough, but science has recently shown us that isn't the case. Research into how our biology makes us bigger is a growing field; factors include the bacteria in our gut and the micro-biome, as well as our genetics and other complex processes still not fully understood. Obesity is also strongly linked to our social circumstances: how much money we earn, how educated we are and where we live.

Here's the thing: obesity for some, not all, is more like a disease with complications than a major character flaw. It's not that people who are overweight lack discipline or self-control; it comes down to a complex interaction of our genetics, our environment, our day-to-day lives and factors we're still learning about. Obesity is not a choice or a screw-up, but rather a disease that carries its own complications, leading to other illnesses. Our bias against obese people is changing, but that still doesn't mean that being obese is good for our health.

What we know for certain is that when we store extra fat, it's not just fat on the outside of our bodies that is problematic. Fat is also stored on our insides. When it accumulates around our vital organs, such as our heart or our kidneys, it causes direct damage. The fat that cradles our kidneys causes high blood pressure and impairs liver function; around our heart it makes us more likely to have a heart attack or heart failure and it makes our body resistant to insulin (leading to diabetes).

Fat also accumulates in the throat, leading to obstructive sleep apnoea – sufferers wake repeatedly through the night with obstructed breathing. This can place enormous strain on the heart and lungs as well as lead to exhaustion during the day. The extra weight places stress on our joints, leaving us at risk of arthritis and other aches and pains. The science linking obesity with heart disease and joint disease is strong and, although it's not the only factor leading to these conditions, the link is irrefutable.

Ironically, we sometimes describe where our fat is stored by different fruit shapes. An 'apple' describes people who carry the bulk of their weight around their mid-section. A 'pear' describes someone whose hips are the site of fat storage. Research has shown that 'apples' are more prone to illness than 'pears'; there seems to be something especially unhealthy about fat stored in and around the organs in our abdomen. This type of fat storage is riskier, particularly for heart disease. Unfortunately, we don't get to choose where we store extra fat; our bodies store it this way due to genetic programming, our diet and levels of hormones such as cortisol and androgens.

Obesity places us at risk of a number of serious, life-changing diseases and forms a part of the metabolic syndrome where we see weight gain (particularly in our midsection), diabetes, high blood pressure, raised cholesterol and what we call impaired fasting glucose, which is like pre-diabetes. We cannot ignore this growing problem: since the 1980s, there has been an extraordinary rise in our weight and the illnesses associated with it. The number of diabetics grew by around 400 per cent from 1980 to 2014, and heart disease is now Australia's leading single cause of death with 18,590 lives lost to it in 2017. In addition, about one-third of the population has high blood pressure and as a result more people are being killed by strokes. This is also happening ever earlier in life.

The reasons include the changing nature of work and demographics of the workforce. More of us are sitting behind a desk all day, rather than walking around a farm or construction site. The dramatic rise in female employment, combined with increasing industrialisation of the food sector, has led to an increase in the consumption of processed and ready-made foods, most of which are far higher in sugar, salt and fat. A recent survey showed 85 per cent of Australians had eaten fast food in the previous six months – the most popular were McDonald's, KFC and Subway. The first McDonald's opened in the Sydney suburb of Yagoona in 1971; in the past twenty years, the total number of fast-food outlets in this country has increased from 12,000 to 1.8 million.

At the same time, longer working hours and lengthy commutes have led to a decline in the time spent on sport and exercise. The most recent Australian Health Survey revealed that only 55 per cent of adults aged 18-64 get the recommended amount of exercise – 150 minutes a week of moderate physical activity. The Australian stereotype of the lean, bronzed digger is decades out of date; we are now the third most obese country in the world.

The stigma of weight

Recently I've noticed a trend, especially among people who are very rightly fighting weight stigma, to make sweeping statements such as 'obesity doesn't cause disease' or 'bias kills people with obesity, not their fat'. I have to challenge that because it ignores a lot of the science at hand. It is absolutely true that as a society and even as health-care professionals, we're horrible to fat people and this has a marked impact on their health. However, there are causative links between obesity, especially the presence of fat in certain areas of our body, and other complications such as diabetes. In diabetes, for example, the fat tissue contributes to insulin resistance as well as possibly the amount of insulin the pancreas produces. Both parts of the science (bias, or psychology, and illness) can be true and we must take them both into account.

Our physical health isn't the only thing at risk. People who are overweight and obese are often subject to discrimination and ridicule. Weight stigma is a risk factor for mental and physical disease in its own right. Research into how fat people get treated in the doctor's surgery has shown that, for instance, they may get less time with a doctor or lower quality medical care. In a number of countries, health-care systems lack the resources of time and adequate numbers of dietitians or exercise programs to give people the tools they need to make positive health changes.

We are mean to fat people. They're very often the basis for comic relief in films and society at large. While it's easy to call obesity a character flaw, the causes are not simple. On one hand, we all make our own food choices and perhaps we eat more than our bodies need. However, those choices do not happen in a vacuum. Obesity happens in a biological context where some people are more prone to weight gain. And food choices happen in environments where we are too often presented with unhealthy foods that are easier to find and cheaper.

Even in a hospital, a place where we're surrounded by illness and people trying to get better, we make it bloody hard to make good food choices. In every hospital I have worked in, the lack of healthy food options is insane. How are health-care workers meant to eat well in this environment? How the hell are the patients, or their visiting support people? One hospital got rid of sugary drinks such as Coke for a short time, but it didn't last because staff and patients alike near-on revolted. More often than not, we're given an abundance of unhealthy choices and the healthy choices are inaccessible or completely absent.

We're wired to want to eat 'tasty' food; our biology encourages us to overindulge in fatty, sugary and salty foods. Soft drinks or sodas give us huge amounts of calories and sugar but no satiety or feeling of fullness. In the US, half of all adults have at least one soda a day, with about 16 teaspoons of sugar in every regular 600 ml bottle. Researchers are exploring the addictive qualities of these types of food, meaning, biologically speaking, the ways in which they act on the brain that could make it harder to give them up. It's a contentious point, and comparing food to substances such as drugs is way too simplistic, but certainly it's an interesting area for research.

Fit and fat?

Is it possible to be fit and fat? There is a group of people who meet the criteria for obesity, yet don't seem to have any nasty side effects such as heart disease or diabetes. The concept has been publicised widely in the media and investigated extensively by researchers. I have heard patients, friends and celebrities say that although they are big they are healthy, or fit, or both.

Most research has called into question 'metabolically healthy obesity', which is how 'fit and fat' is described in scientific journals. The bulk of the research shows us some crucial points. Firstly, obesity is just one aspect of health and an overall assessment. That's to say, you can't judge a book by its cover. Just by looking at someone's weight in isolation doesn't tell you how healthy or unhealthy they are; that is true for people who are bigger and those who are smaller. (For children, this may be even more relevant. Some claim we place far too much emphasis on a child's weight and body size and not enough on their overall physical, cognitive and psychosocial growth and development.)

Health is associated with our weight, but also other factors such as how active we are, what we eat, whether we smoke and our genetics. Our fitness is one factor that could offset the effects of our lifestyle or size, and can help us to be 'fit and fat'. At present, researchers have largely reported that we don't know enough about this condition. Research published in powerhouse medical journals shows that if you follow these 'fit but fat' people over a decade, despite the fact they were once healthy and obese, they don't always stay that way. Many go on to develop complications of their obesity, maybe indicating a loss of fitness and healthy behaviours, or the natural course of their body weight.

That's not to say so-called 'fit and fat' people aren't out there. There is probably a small number who seem to be naturally predisposed to avoid some of the complications of obesity. It is likely their healthy lifestyle offers some protection. Although obesity is one piece of the puzzle in determining health, it is not the only one.

Fat on the inside

While we might think that being a normal or healthy weight protects us from illness, it isn't always the case. Studies of people with diabetes show that 15–20 per cent are of normal body weight. These people are more likely to be male, not be active enough, smoke, or store their fat in those central, danger areas. Sometimes they are referred to as 'thin outside, fat inside' to hammer home their health battle. It's estimated that 20 per cent of the population, despite being of normal weight, are at risk of illnesses we normally associate with obesity. This is one area where BMI falls flat.

BMI measurements certainly have their limitations. BMI doesn't tell us where the weight is stored or what it's made up of. A heavy body builder with huge amounts of muscle would have a falsely high BMI. A tall person, who isn't what we might call overweight based on their appearance, may store their fat in their abdomen, around their organs. One study demonstrated that one in three adults has their health misclassified by BMI. That's not to say the calculation was wrong. Some skinny people had metabolic evidence of health issues, such as high cholesterol or high blood glucose, while some bigger people had metabolic evidence of being healthy. And, although a lot of research has shown a connection between

BMI and disease, there have been studies over the years that have gone against the trend. Some have shown that more body weight actually makes us more likely to survive some diseases; for example, certain cancers. Obesity experts are quick to point out that this has not been proven to the point where we should ignore the health effects of extra weight. The 'Obesity Paradox' does not mean that extra weight is actually beneficial, but rather that BMI tells only part of a person's health story.

BMI is a screening tool; if you score close to either end of the scale, rather than being told categorically that this makes you unhealthy, it should primarily trigger more investigation. A large study published in the *Journal of the American College of Cardiology* showed a relationship between BMI and heart disease in a group of people followed for many years. Dismissing everything we know about the associations between obesity and certain illnesses just because BMI is a flawed tool seems like throwing the baby out with the bathwater.

Obesity is a constant public health pressure and, we're told, a growing burden on society. However, some argue that the way we talk about it makes it harder to manage; I tend to agree. I am yet to meet a patient who is obese and unaware of it. I can see the shame on their face whenever it comes up. Constant messages that being fat is bad for you reduce public sympathy and lead to stigma that might stop people seeking help. Researchers from Swinburne University even argue that calling obesity an epidemic is harmful, because it might place further emphasis on the idea that health equates to being skinny, further fuelling the obsession with body appearance rather than body health. Our obsession with being skinny could be leading to growing rates of body dissatisfaction.

I acknowledge that it is uncomfortable to talk about our weight. It is a source of shame for people of all shapes and sizes. Weight bias absolutely impacts on the health of people who are bigger, and health-care workers contribute to this as much as the general population. I have heard colleagues call overweight people 'fatties' or make jokes. It's inappropriate and unprofessional and causes untold damage to health and wellbeing. However, just because we've long been cruel and dismissive of people who are overweight and we've caused harm in that process does not mean we need to stop talking about it. There are doctors and patients alike who advocate eliminating the word 'obesity' from our vocabulary because it causes embarrassment, bias and ill health.

In 2018, the Australian government released findings of a parliamentary enquiry into the so-called 'obesity epidemic'. One of the recommendations was to fight stigma, and one way to do that was to stop using the word obesity in health promotion and prevention programs. They conceded that there isn't an alternative for 'obesity' in medical settings or policy naming yet. While the term 'fat' is used by some groups to reclaim what they're called by others (following other social justice movements) that word might not suit everyone so, for now, we look for a more encompassing, less stigmatising term.

There is a tendency to blame the individual for the fact that they are bigger, especially if they're unhealthy. While we send messages that it's not okay to be fat, we also support a society that advertises junk food to kids. Think of the hypocrisy of the hospital whose staff berate patients for not eating well, but only offer hot chips and Coke for lunch! UK research has revealed that among the many causes of obesity, very little has to do with willpower or personal responsibility. If we want to tackle obesity, we need to empower people to make good choices, not let them flounder in a hospital food court of bad choices.

Sitting: the new smoking?

Linked to the fact that we're getting bigger, of course, is the fact that we're also doing a lot less physical activity. Headlines like 'Sitting is the new smoking' indicate the huge threat inactivity poses to our health. We have long known the value of moving our bodies: the Greeks and Romans celebrated a strong and healthy body, and early physicians promoted exercise as a magic pill. Something has gone awry, however, with a recent study finding that globally 5.3 million people a year are estimated to die from inactivity. Lack of movement has been tied to many diseases, including heart disease and dementia; being active makes a big dent in our risk of diabetes, heart disease, joint problems and premature death.

Despite the fact that most countries have joined the World Health Organization's (WHO) commitment to get people more active, it's not really working. Public health campaigns may be missing the mark, or the barriers to exercise might be simply still too strong. We appear to even be going backwards. In Australia, 56 per cent of adults are not active enough, and that becomes 66 per cent for women from a low-socioeconomic background. Elderly people are also not active enough, with serious repercussions for their health and ability to recover from disease. These statistics are echoed in many countries around the world. For entertainment, we watch an average of 13 hours of television per week and now spend almost seven hours a day accessing the internet via computers, tablets and phones. Even children as young as two years old are notching up 90 minutes of television a day. We commute in our cars, driving 17,600 minutes a year. An Australian study showed that commuting more than an hour a day by car increased the risk of ill health.

Women's inactivity deserves particular attention. A survey of American women showed that just 19 per cent meet the guidelines for aerobic and strength training, meaning the majority are missing out on the extensive benefits of exercise. An Australian study reported that physical activity falls during girlhood and by age 24 over half of women have stopped playing sport. Reasons include lack of time or a safe space, or lack of access. Overcoming stereotypes that women shouldn't play sport, or feeling self-conscious while being active are also disincentives to regular exercise. We're giving women mixed advice – exercise, but make sure you look good doing it – and this is costing lives.

Despite a huge commitment from public health organisations like WHO and the backing of governments around the world, we're not winning. Even when research has shown the success of a particular study aimed at increasing activity, it tends to fail the real-world test by not working when it's scaled up. Given that the problem of inactivity spans our whole lives and affects virtually every aspect of our daily routine, it will take more than just creating more parks or getting kids to play during school lunch. Every sector of the public and private spheres, including our workplaces, needs to commit to change, if we're ever going to improve. Even though we are fully aware of the gravity of the problem, we don't appear to be getting any closer to solving it.

The food wars

What we eat plays a huge role in how healthy we are, of course, but unfortunately the thriving science of nutrition is a growing target for pseudoscientific 'influencers' and commercial entities. Social media is filled with cries of 'Food is medicine' and 'Every time you eat, you're fighting disease or feeding it', in an attempt to illustrate the importance of good food. Even though nutrition is an easy target for bogus advice, it is also crucial to health. Changes in science or conflicting advice make it harder for us to follow a healthy way of eating.

Sayings such 'you are what you eat' or 'an apple a day keeps the doctor away' are part of conventional wisdom. Incidentally, that old saying about eating apples probably does hold some weight. A study of more than 8000 people published in the *Journal of the American Medical Association* showed that regularly eating apples leads to lower rates of medication prescriptions – not because apples are powerful disease fighters, but because regular fruit eaters probably eat pretty well most of the time. Even while debate has raged about what we should or shouldn't eat, the importance of good food is well known; we generally understand the link between diet and certain diseases such as obesity and high blood pressure.

But rather than stick with that easy-to-understand old advice, we have made things ever more complicated. Instead of 'eat more vegetables', we are now told which vegetable, where to buy it, whether it should be organic, and how we should cook and serve it to maximise its benefits. We have taken 'an apple a day' and turned it into 'an apple is high in flavonoids which fight cancer' – a gross overstatement. It is challenging enough to keep up with the basics of good diet, let alone these layers of complexity.

Despite that, we keep trying. We are more and more obsessed with what we eat, what we read and what we do. We're tracking macros and reading food labels and are discerning consumers in the quest for cleaner, leaner bodies. Restaurants and food chains now claim to be 'healthy' and menu items are prefaced with words such as 'super', 'green' or 'clean'. We are presented with a list of popular ingredients all designed to make our insides better than ever before, coming off the back of public interest in healthy guts or metabolism boosting.

Food is central to our wellbeing, but which foods are best for us has been hotly contested, particularly in the last few years. Decades ago, nutritional guidelines called for low-fat, high-carbohydrate approaches, emphasising grains and refuting the health benefits of foods such as eggs and nuts. However, as nutrition science evolves, scientific researchers and the person in the street have become more interested in optimal eating. Once thought to be 'not so bad', sugar has been declared by some as public enemy number one and fats appear to be having their moment in the sun. Former nutritional pariahs such as nuts and avocados are back on people's healthy menus. No single substance is responsible for all our ill health, nor is one particular food its panacea. Demonising sugar, for example, is unhelpful, firstly because it damages our relationship with food and leads to guilt, but most importantly because it fails to acknowledge the complexity of food, nutrition and disease.

The constant changing opinion of what's good and what's bad seems to have led to distrust in nutritional research. Compounding this is the fact that 'big food' sponsors a number of research projects or lobbies for food information to be presented to the public in a commercial context. The public understands this potential conflict of interest and this breeds suspicion. For example, Australian foods carry a 'Health Star Rating', which came under fire when consumers and experts noticed high nutritional ratings – 3.5 out of 5 stars – being given to sugary foods. This is obviously misleading to the public and the undue influence of the food industry was blamed.

This distrust of experts has opened the door for dozens of people with very little in the way of health or nutritional knowledge to share their beliefs online and gain huge followings. The rise of 'superfoods', such as kale, coconut oil and quinoa, has coincided with pseudoscience around them, often disseminated on social media and popular blogs and websites. These foods, despite having no major advantage over cheaper, more readily-available healthy foods, have seen a surge in popularity.

Will the real experts please stand up?

As public appetite grows for finding the 'secret' foods that lead to health, so too has the number of books, documentaries and blogs claiming to have uncovered the truth about foods and nutrition. Some of the biggest nutrition-related books in recent years have been written by journalists or full-time writers, which begs the question, where are the qualified experts? Why aren't they using their expertise to explain what's good for us?

The recommendations of popular nutrition superstars have come under fire for being unscientific or unattainable to most people. Coconut oil, for example, was touted as a panacea just a few years ago, yet research has called its benefits into question; in some cases, it can be shown to be detrimental to health. Yet it's still promoted by social media darlings as the secret to health or dietary success. In some cases, popular bloggers have risked lives by stating that they can cure cancer, leading to growing numbers of people completely shunning conventional, proven treatment.

Nutrition science is complicated research to conduct. Although we want to look at a particular type of fat, humans don't eat single nutrients; we eat food, so the effect of a particular nutrient can be hard to separate. And when we research people's diets, we often rely heavily on their recall or self-reported eating, which I'm sure we can all understand is not ideal. This kind of research also takes time and doesn't give us the instant answers we all want. How often have you thrown your hands in the air and said, 'Wait, I thought that was bad for us?' as the list of foods we're supposed to be in love with changes?

Regardless, food is vital to our wellbeing as individuals, a society and even to our planet. Our complicated relationships with food have led to a state where food has become our undoing but has the power to be our salvation. Despite what the diet industry would have you believe, it probably has very little to do with surefire meal plans, superfoods or one eating plan being superior to the other. What we eat does not need to be complicated and it should happen in an environment where it is easy to be healthy and harder to be the opposite.

Malnourished and overweight

In modern society vast numbers of us suffer from illnesses relating to the overconsumption of food, or excess food of low nutritional value. Yet, at the same time, huge numbers of people globally remain hungry or undernourished. Malnutrition used to mean famine. Nowadays a malnourished child could present as underweight *or* overweight, and there are plenty of adults who are overweight or obese *and* malnourished. A lack of healthy food has led to people missing out on nutrients, such as iron and zinc, which are vital for our red blood cells and immune system and for reducing the risk of heart disease and diabetes. It's not just our physical wellbeing at risk: malnutrition contributes to differences in educational attainment, female empowerment and poverty.

In the past few decades our diet has changed to include increased amounts of sugar-sweetened beverages and processed foods containing trans fats and high-fructose corn syrup. Many people also eat bigger portions and rely on ready-made or restaurant meals of variable quality. The Australian Bureau of Statistics data shows that Australians consume an average of 14 teaspoons of sugar a day, with 14–18-year-old boys having a whopping 38 teaspoons per day. WHO guidelines recommend no more than six teaspoons a day. Australians consume 81 per cent of their sugar from nutrient-poor soft drinks and processed snacks.

Most trans fats are formed through an industrial process popular with manufacturers because it extends the shelf life of foods. These fats have been identified as so dangerous to health that seven European countries have banned them, with many more asking manufacturers to limit their use. Trans fats not only promote weight gain, they also appear to cause damage to our heart and blood vessels and promote diseases such as diabetes. If trans fats were medicine, they would never be approved for human consumption.

Foods laden with trans fats or sugars are also thought to trigger reactions in the body that promote illness and dysfunction. They alter where we store fat, contribute to a fatty liver and increase our amounts of LDL, or bad cholesterol. They also cause inflammation of many of the body's organs, including the gut and blood vessels, which can act as a precursor to disease.

The popularity of these foods has much to do with marketing, especially to children. Research has shown that virtually all of the foods marketed to children exceed the recommended intakes of calories or sugar they should eat to maintain health. These foods are also cheap and quick to prepare, increasing their appeal to time-poor, low-income families. And with high fat and sugar levels, the food is often very tasty, adding to its general appeal. But altering this is a challenge – eating food is a social act and changing our nutrition can mean changing social structures and practices.

Disordered eating

At the same time as we're eating too much – too much food overall or too much unhealthy food – eating disorders are on the rise. These include conditions such as anorexia nervosa, bulimia nervosa, binge-eating disorder and others. We're also seeing growth in what is termed 'disordered eating', when a person's food intake is not quite right for their body or they have incredibly restrictive eating patterns that threaten their physical and mental wellbeing. This group of eating disorders doesn't quite meet the criteria for one of the main disorders, but could be surprisingly common.

It's been estimated that around 15 per cent of Australian women will experience an eating disorder at some point during their life; a further 20 per cent will suffer with an undiagnosed eating disorder. These figures have been rising, and there has also been an increase in diagnoses in young men. Sufferers face serious risks to their physical health and increased rates of suicide. They can sometimes struggle to access appropriate treatment because their symptoms are either unrecognised or too complicated for our health systems to deal with. Despite this, hospital admissions for eating disorders in the UK continue to grow, nearly doubling between 2010 and 2017. A 2012 report estimated that treating eating disorders cost the Australian health system $100 million. Anorexia is our deadliest mental disorder, with an estimated mortality rate of 20 per cent.

The causes of eating disorders include genetic factors, psychological and personality traits, and life events such as childhood abuse. However, how we view our own bodies is also affected by the media, society and our peers. People who have recovered from eating disorders are rightly critical of the way we glamourise dieting and thinness by valuing being thin at any cost – something that normalises disordered and highly restrictive eating. If it yields the desired results, the health costs are simply ignored. As the incredibly damaging saying goes: 'You can never be too rich or too thin.'

Smokes and booze

Despite many years of health warnings, we still smoke and drink to excess. Tobacco use remains one of the leading causes of death around the world and is a risk factor for lung cancer, bladder cancer, emphysema, heart attacks, strokes, and peripheral vascular disease – people literally lose their legs for a smoke. Excessive alcohol use leads to cancers and liver dysfunction as well as increasing our chances of being involved in an accident. Despite restrictions on both of these commonly used drugs, and knowledge of the risks, young people still take up smoking, while binge drinking is a public health nightmare.

Women in particular tend to smoke for stress relief and, worryingly, they are more likely to take up smoking as a form of weight control. Women are 31 per cent less likely to quit successfully than men. So, despite the fact that smoking is socially unacceptable and unhealthy, this is trumped in some cases by concern over appearance.

Pretty unhealthy

If illness rates keep increasing, we are all in a lot of trouble. Our health systems will struggle to keep up, but there are other far-reaching consequences. In 2017 life expectancy in the US fell for the third year in a row and we could start to see that happening all around the world. People might continue to live a long time, but in poorer quality health. On a bad day at work, with increasingly younger and sicker people, I feel like I'm losing the fight against ballooning rates of disease.

The reasons for this are everywhere. We live in a world that has created a perfect storm of commercial interests, imperfect community interventions, economic disadvantage, inactivity, too much unhealthy food, a persistent tobacco industry, and excessive use of alcohol. Our society pays heavily for this unhealthy way of life but pays very little to prevent it. For those of us who are in some way connected with the lifestyle diseases, personally or professionally, it is a soul-destroying battle.

We have completely lost sight of what health truly is. Our systems are broken and I worry that we are image obsessed rather than health obsessed. It means we take on a relentless and challenging pursuit of looking a certain way in the hope that it will bring us health. It won't; it is just complicating an already complex problem and making it sometimes impossibly hard to do what's actually good for us.

The illnesses that now take years off our lives and the life out of our years can be prevented, halted or at the very least slowed down, but that is going to take a new approach. One that cuts the ties linking beauty with health and unattractiveness with disease. A new approach will have to disregard the false hopes, unrealistic expectations, bad science, stigma and unkindness, replacing them with achievable goals, strong science and compassion. In order to be healthier, we need to re-examine every aspect of our lives.

Chapter 2

WHY WORKING OUT ISN'T WORKING OUT

'Excuses don't burn calories.'

UNKNOWN

I went shopping a few weeks ago. I'd had a busy and frustrating week and hadn't exercised as much as I'd wanted so I was feeling a bit out of sorts. I walked past the sports store, went inside and bought a pair of running tights that I liked but which, apparently, also had the added benefit of motivating me. I thought to myself that I would absolutely want to exercise that evening because I had a new exercise outfit, and who doesn't want to take something new for a spin?

I stopped this train of thought: it made no sense. Where did that kind of disordered thinking come from? I was angry at myself for being sucked in to what is simply marketing. Even if my new tights made me go for a run that evening, they would almost certainly lose some of their magic touch after the first wear.

Over the years, my personal motivations for exercising or eating well have ranged from the advertising at the sports store to fitting into a particular piece of clothing. Such as the 'skinny shorts' I had purchased as a 15-year-old and deluded my 29-year-old self into considering a worthy goal. I ate well and exercised to improve my physical and mental health, to look like one of the women on *Bikini Body Guide*-creator and personal trainer Kayla Itsines' Instagram, or to avoid having to be operated on by one of my colleagues for heart disease. There was the time I thought I just needed to be healthier – and that was a specific number on a scale that I was running and dieting to achieve.

Everywhere we turn, something is supposedly trying to make us healthier. We appear to be falling all over ourselves to eat healthy, look healthy, dress healthy and perhaps be healthy. The ways in which we're embarking on this quest seem to fill an inordinate amount of conversations and probably an excessive amount of our private inside thoughts and to-do lists. We're in overdrive in our quest to be the healthiest and best versions of ourselves.

We cover our bodies in activewear, and on our wrists we sport wearable technology to log how active we have been that day. T-shirts with slogans like 'Sweat is Just Fat Crying' or the more inspirational 'Never Ever Give Up' are the wardrobe du jour. Stores sell activewear in all styles, shapes and colours designed to make us look our best while being active fills every shopping centre. There are gyms every few doors along the street and they're open 24 hours a day so there is never any excuse for missing a workout.

Our step goals or exercise goals, once attained, flash on digital screens as a virtual pat on the back for another step towards conquering those skinny jeans that are a little too snug.

We participate in exercise programs and challenges with virtual trophies or actual prizes, rewarding the outstanding physical commitment to a gym's latest challenge. Challenge to what? To be our best selves, or some similar ideology? We wear tops emblazoned with our latest challenge, an obstacle course or our boutique gym, as proud as an Olympic medal.

Our medicine cabinets have been replaced with supplement cabinets as we stock up on vitamins and minerals to give us better skin, nails, guts and to help burn calories. (Listen closely and you might even hear fat cells screaming.) We wear sunscreen every day to avoid premature ageing, and use organic oils to make our skin glow with health.

Our Instagram feeds feature photos of buddha bowls, farmer's markets vegetables (organic, of course) and smoothies sipped in the sunshine, while holding a yoga pose. Our smiling faces are captioned with inspirational celebrity quotes. We read self-help books giving techniques for emotional wellbeing or a dedicated number of steps to manage our weight.

We are, seemingly, living our best lives. We are so health-conscious, it permeates every single aspect of our day. Everything we do is geared towards being the 'best version of ourselves'. And, yet, as often as we are presented with health, we are also confronted with ill health. Am I imagining all of this healthiness?

While we might be living longer, those extra years, according to news stories on the latest research, are filled with more illness than ever. A growing body of research shows we're getting fatter, eating more, exercising less, while at the same time suffering with anxiety, depression and eating disorders.

Adrift, in a sea of activewear: what are we doing to be healthy?

Gyms are big business. When you look around and see gyms everywhere, you're not imagining it. They have been opening at a rapid rate in what is really just a short period of time. From 2012, in just three short years, the number of gyms in the United States grew by 5,500 to a staggering 36,180.

That increase has been repeated around the world, in Canada, Latin America, Europe and Australia. In my early twenties, I would drive 20 minutes to get to the gym and there really weren't many people there. Nowadays, I have three separate gyms, two Pilates studios and a yoga studio within ten minutes' walk from my house. And if you feel like a 4am workout, 24-hour gyms are now the standard. Opened due to the demand for flexible workout hours, they now make up a large number of gyms around the world.

And we're joining these gyms in droves. Since the early 2000s, the number of members has soared, nearly doubling in the US. Which, with an average spend of $US 800 annually, is not an inexpensive exercise. Similarly, in Australia and the UK, millions of people have gym memberships.

Traditional gyms are also being challenged by specialised workouts such as CrossFit, which are now as universal as fast food chains. Established in 2000, CrossFit has expanded from the US to become a worldwide phenomenon. CNBC's article on the ubiquity of CrossFit reports that there are thousands of CrossFit gyms (or boxes as they're known) in over 120 countries and the cult-like workout boasts millions of devotees.

Despite all these gyms and all these members, a large proportion of people don't use their memberships. In 2016, *USA Today* reported that 67 per cent of gym memberships go unused. An Australian report states that Australians waste $AU 1.8 billion a year on unused gym memberships. (I finally cancelled mine last week after leaving it unused for months.) The eye-watering part of this tale is the financial gain of these companies with reported revenues of $US 30 billion in 2017. This industry has seen incredible growth every year with no signs of slowing down.

The diet industry goes hand in hand with wanting to be healthy. A little like gyms, new diets are everywhere and it seems as though everyone is 'on a diet', a 'detox' or a 'cleanse' at one time or another. There are literally dozens of different regimes to follow, from low-carbohydrate to highly restrictive diets like the Cabbage Soup Diet. Estimates suggest that 45 million Americans go on a diet every year with a stunning 45 per cent of New Year's Resolutions being directed at losing weight. According to the National Eating Disorders Association, 58.6 per cent of girls and 28.2 per cent of boys are actively dieting at any time.

Old-school diet companies such as Weight Watchers (now called WW to take the emphasis off weight/pull the wool over our eyes) have maintained a huge market share in what is a $US 175 billion industry. Even with bad publicity for diets and shifts away from traditional commercial diets, the industry is going to continue to make money from our desire to get healthy, slim or better-looking. Resounding celebrity endorsements such as those from Oprah Winfrey, Kate Hudson (who is still probably smaller than most women) and DJ Khaled backing Weight Watchers, and the persistent growth of lifestyle diseases, are keeping diets firmly in the health picture.

Alongside commercial products and programs, the diet book industry is an enormous force. Pretty much every bestseller list has an abundance of diet and health books in its ranks. Even well-known chefs such as Jamie Oliver have released recipe books with new-and-improved, healthy takes on family favourites. Around 5 million diet books are sold in the US each year.

For those who choose to shun diets in favour of 'healthy eating' or 'clean eating', the growth in these approaches to health, weight loss or general wellbeing continue to grow in popularity. Clean eating can attribute a large amount of its success to social media, where users mark their healthy meals with the hashtag #cleaneating. On Instagram alone, the #cleaneating hashtag features tens of millions of posts.

Clean eating is also joined by an ever-growing number of diets and eating plans. Dietary plans such as gluten-free, ketogenic, low-carb, alkaline or detox diets join the ranks of plans promising to help us meet our goals. We're also becoming savvier about what foods we eat, looking to fulfil high-protein or low-sugar goals. It seems we can't seem to resist the allure of healthy labels. More people are buying foods labelled high-protein, low-sugar, organic or gluten-free. And, despite being largely unnecessary or disproven to aid health for a large number of people, dietary supplements also continue to rake in our hard-earned cash.

Technology is another area where we're putting our time and money to reach our goals. Smartphone app stores such as Apple AppStore and Android Marketplace are filled with apps designed to help us plan and track our diet or exercise. We can watch every scrap of food we eat, every step we take and every minute we spend asleep. Forty per cent of Americans use fitness and tracking apps and spend over a billion dollars each year for the privilege. Millions of devices such as FitBits are sold and each iteration of the popular yet very expensive Apple Watch promises even more tech to keep us in tip-top shape.

Of course, to do all this, we need to look good and that has seen an explosion in sportswear, activewear and athleisure. From the days of just a handful of traditional retailers such as Nike or Adidas, now there are dozens of sportswear retailers in store or online. Even conventional designers and retailers are getting in on the act, launching their own sportswear lines. And we are buying the hell out of it. *Forbes* magazine puts revenue from activewear in the billions, with no signs of slowing down. Even cosmetics companies are cashing in, with launches of waterproof and sweatproof sports make-up increasingly available.

And to look for inspiration for our healthy lives, we follow every movement of social media influencers, such as fitness model Michelle Lewin, fellow fitness model Jen Selter and Kayla Itsines. These three women have millions of followers between them. Itsines alone sees thousands of new followers each day. With posts on their diets, exercise and a spattering of motivational quotes, these big-name fitness influencers inspire and educate millions on how to attain their goals. But more on them later.

Here's the upshot to all of these facts and figures. They are not health. They are not even close to being indicators of what health is. We look at the number of people joining gyms, wearing sneakers or even buying diet books and say, we have to be getting healthier. Look at all of the time, money and brain power that people spend on their health.

Except of course, these statistics are all an illusion.

Confused? I am. Despite the fact that we know more than ever about health and disease, it seems to be a losing battle. All the time, money and thought that we're expending in this so-called war seems to be making us sicker and poorer. In fact, this is often how our quest to be healthy is described: battles with bulges and wars on waistlines.

You, healthier?

We might say we've signed up to a gym to be healthy. But can we really say what health is? When asked, maybe we'd say that being healthy is not having any disease. Or that it's being slim or being able to run a certain distance or simply feeling good. Our definition of health probably varies depending on who we are. A young woman conscious of the way her body looks might call it being a certain weight, whereas someone with an illness, say cancer, would call being healthy a scan that shows their chemotherapy is working.

WHO originally defined health as a 'state of complete physical, mental, and social wellbeing'. This has been debated and expanded to encompass a number of things, including the ability to bounce back from illness and the actions you take in life to maintain this health. The thing I like about this definition and find important is that our health is contingent on its being complete. It's about the physical body, mental wellbeing and even society being healthy too. Please make note that nowhere does this definition mention fitting into a dress.

Our modern obsession with health has moved away from this scientific definition and towards something that can be the basis for more sinister ideas. 'Healthism' was originally coined by Robert Crawford in 1980; he defined it as a preoccupation with personal health as the primary focus and achievement of wellbeing. Crawford was particularly critical of the way healthism places both the blame and solution for ill-health on the individual, rather than the unbelievably complex interaction of factors that make us healthy or not. Basically, if you're sick, it's your own fault.

Healthism has also evolved to be a moral judgement, so if you're not utterly and totally dedicated to your health, you're a failure as a human. Health is now advertised as a project, a need to be the most beautiful, glowing, energetic and best version of yourself, preferably documented on social media in a carefully cultivated series of squares demonstrating your physical, emotional and moral superiority. Popular health advocates aren't commonly those admitting to being well-rounded and flawed; they're more likely to be modelesque people who talk vaguaries about minerals and meditation and savasana.

Health has become wrapped up in profit and bad policies, pseudoscience and fashion. Rather than using the concerning unhealthy future that faces us as a reason to scientifically, compassionately and responsibly restore health, it's used as a basis for greed and bullying. A whole industry has grown in recent years that capitalises on our fear – a fear of being unhealthy – which so often masquerades as fear of not being 'enough'. Not skinny enough, not popular enough and not attractive enough.

Exactly how sick does our world need to be before we stop paying attention to pseudoscience, beauty and profit? It is long overdue that we do something real about it, because doling out advice such as 'eat less', 'be thin' or 'work out' isn't working.

To truly tackle the health of our society, we need to start looking at the realities of health. We need to place emphasis where it is going to work and that emphasis is not on making us look better. Health is about us being wholly better. Illness is not pretty, but that doesn't mean that our health is beauty. Unhooking the obsession we have with health being beauty will allow us to stop being swept up by all the things that are not good for our health, and start fighting back in this war on disease.

I picked up a magazine in a petrol station a while ago because I saw the headline saying: 'You, healthier' and I wondered what the hell that actually meant. After reading the article, I'm not sure I'm any wiser. It was laden with vague references to health and was heavy on fad diets and popular workouts. The idea that we can achieve health by engaging in specific but fashionable behaviours is being pushed to the forefront of our minds. I spent $8 on this magazine that provided me with a vague list of diets and exercise regimens to follow and asked the important question if I could be truly fit and healthy without doing HIIT (high-intensity interval training). I flicked to the page of the workout promising to burn fat like 'no other workout could' and laughed out loud as I saw the same exercises my dad used to perform 30 years ago from his *Arnold Schwarzenegger's Body Building* book. None of this is new, nor is it the magic pill to a healthier you that it claims to be.

Granted, the concept of health as defined by WHO is a bit nebulous. But we're not being given the truth when we are told directly or indirectly that healthy means washboard abs, yoga pants, green smoothies or a perfect Instagram picture. We're looking for something concrete to define and give us health. Is it any wonder we're aimlessly jumping from trend to trend, gym to

CrossFit and spending our hard-earned cash on things we don't enjoy or, in the realm of vitamins and supplements, that don't even work? The problem is they're a shiny substitute at best and plain old marketing at worst and I call bullshit.

Health is a vast concept. It's the WHO definition and it's much more. For me, it's my blood pressure returning to normal levels and my mental stress being at a manageable level. It's being able to prevent the preventable diseases and live a life that is meaningful and social. It's being loved and loving others. Health is the health of my community and my planet. It's an effective and equitable health-care system that treats all people with compassion.

What motivates you?

As I was in the queue at the supermarket, fresh from my annoyance at the health magazine experience, I examined all the magazine covers. In particular, I studied the many health magazines. The covers seemed to scream, urging me to 'take action' towards a healthy lifestyle, or a 'perfect weight' or a certain number of weeks to my best body ever. I could even join the 'fast track to my perfect body'. They appeared as turbo-charged motivations towards a better, healthier self, superimposed over the image of a model or actress with a seemingly flawless body.

I could see the motivation leaping off the covers, nearly shouting at me to buy the hero food or get the summer 'bikini body'. I started to wonder whether it's in motivation, though, that we all get tripped up. Despite our best intentions, or the catch cries of magazines or fitness influencers on social media, what gets us exercising or eating right can actually backfire.

Now it's reasonable to assume that most people have heard exercise and healthy food are good for us. Motivation is one of the key things that will help us to start engaging in healthy behaviours and keep them up, and there has been a fair amount of research done to see what motivates people in these areas. While many want to lose weight for health goals, such as a recent diagnosis of high blood pressure, or to improve longevity, one of the biggest reasons is to look better. People with obesity list this 66 per cent of the time; those without obesity list it 59 per cent of the time.

There is a theory of motivation called self-determination, which is thought to be important in the motivation to be healthy. It's a set of three basic psychological needs that have to be met in order to maintain motivation. They are competence, autonomy and connectedness to other people. If we can do exercise that taps into these basic psychological needs, it's thought much more likely we

---

What is self-determination theory?

Self-determination theory was first described by Edward Deci and Richard Ryan in the 1970s, and is a psychological theory all about motivation. The theory looks at internal versus external motivators and the social and cultural factors that contribute to or oppose our motivation, our wellbeing and how well we do a task. This theory says that motivators that foster our **autonomy**, our **competence** and our **relatedness** are the most high-quality motivators. The theory has been applied to pretty much anything you can think of from exercise, to study.

will have self-determination and be able to carry on in our task with a sense of purpose and motivation.

Competence, or being able to master a skill, is something we can all relate to. It would be pretty normal to want to give up an exercise if we weren't good at it, or perhaps we wouldn't cook healthy food if the kitchen is not our strength. We all want to feel we can develop some skill in something, that we've got it down pat. If we feel like we're not good at a sport, or any other skill, we may well give it up.

The autonomy factor is important, because it looks at our empowerment. For instance, if I felt an external pressure from someone telling me to exercise but it wasn't something I really felt I wanted to do, that doesn't empower me or give me any autonomy. If I don't really connect with wanting or needing to do something, I might not do it.

Being supported, particularly by people close to you or by a health-care professional who has your best interests at heart, allows you that opportunity to flourish. We need to get some sort of connectedness from our exercise and that can come in the form of working out in a group, with a trainer or simply by telling others about your achievements or experience, preferably family and friends rather than social media, where it's pretty fashionable to document your workout for likes.

In addition, we can look at whether motivation comes from outside (extrinsic) or within (intrinsic). An extrinsic motivator might be fitting into an outfit or looking better for a school reunion. It's an outside demand or perhaps a reward that keeps us going. Many of us will think: yes, done that. Studies have shown that half of the information presented in health magazines targeting women is done so in a way that emphasises appearance.

Intrinsic motivation isn't quite so tangible. It's a sense of internal satisfaction or enjoyment derived from doing something. Internally derived motivators tap into our autonomy, which we value very highly according to psychological research. It can also come from altruism: doing something for the good of someone else.

Extrinsic goals don't help us grow as people; intrinsic motivators, on the other hand, can help us grow and evolve if they are helpful to us. Which means we're more likely to sustain that behaviour.

When we exercise or eat well for an external pressure, such as getting into a wedding dress or skinny shorts, we might be able to sustain it for a period of time, but if we feel we're fulfilling a goal for something or someone else then it might not tap into that self-determination. Some research shows that when we're motivated by this kind of external reward, we're more likely to have periods of bingeing if we're on a diet, and more likely to engage in diet behaviours that are actually bad for our health. And, if we're motivated by our appearance, we're actually less likely to participate in physical activity. We seem to work out more when we're proud of our bodies, their fitness and what they can do, rather than how beautiful we think they are.

Another study looked at what motivated people to exercise, focusing on joining a gym versus playing sport. People motivated by external factors such as appearance were more likely to exercise at a gym and this affected their ability to stick at it. They gave up more frequently than people who played sport. Those who played sport seemed to be motivated by enjoyment derived from the game or socialisation – a motivator that might keep people coming back. A similar association has been seen with cardio and gym workouts. Those who participate in cardio (walking, swimming, jogging) seem to derive more personal satisfaction and better body image than gym goers; this again might be about the motivation at play.

What all this means is that when we're dieting or exercising to meet a reward, for example, looking like the woman on Instagram, it can backfire. I imagine this as our bodies being wired to know that health does not equal beauty. Exercising to meet an external goal doesn't necessarily keep us coming back for more. Eating to get a bikini body might work for a while but, soon enough, our motivation and willpower fails us and we slip back into our old ways, bringing the physical changes and emotional distress with it.

This isn't as simple as us failing. The fact that external motivators that don't help us grow are so prevalent is, in part, a marketing game. These beautiful bodies or attractive catch cries appear to be motivating us to pursue health, but the cynic in me thinks they're just trying to sell magazines, diets, gym memberships or gain social media followers. It's sceptical, I know, but since we're shelling out all this cash and spending time doing things that are clearly not working, something is obviously not right. The sooner we can learn to motivate ourselves from the inside, the better it will be for our health.

Does this mean it's bad to want to work out or eat well to look better? As long as we take part in healthy behaviours, does it really matter what starts them or keeps them going? Professor Cecilie Thøgersen-Ntoumani, a psychologist from the Curtin University Physical Activity and Well-Being Lab, is pragmatic about it: it's not realistic to ignore this kind of motivation because it is prevalent and will continue to be so. However, she doesn't necessarily think it's helpful because it may falter in the long run and these motivators are unrealistic and unachievable for a lot of us.

Beauty: not what it seems

Strongly associating health with appearance can be a recipe for disaster in motivating us to be healthy. Beauty is equated with health, but even beauty isn't what it seems. Have you seen that quote? That even the girl in the magazine doesn't look like the girl in the magazine? In a time when everything is air-brushed and edited, the goals we're being presented with are not just unhelpful or unattainable, they're not even real.

It's a bit of a given that images we see in magazines and TV ads are altered. To start with, there is a person who probably has some degree of genetic blessing, whose job it is to be beautiful, who puts time and effort into that the way the rest of us do at work, and who is then made up by teams of professional hair and make-up experts. They're lit and posed or moved in a way that is most flattering for them. In post-production, everything is tidied up to look as perfect as possible, sometimes making bodies and faces unrecognisable. And this is something we're supposed to aspire to? Without a glam squad or professional retouching or the genetics of a model, how is this achievable for most of us?

Actor Rob McElhenny posted a picture of his own body transformation to his Instagram account, showing a bloated tummy turning into the muscular physique many men aspire to. McElhenny was brutally honest in describing the exercise and diet regime that cut out 'everything you like', and workouts six days a week with a trainer who worked on *Magic Mike*. Also, he didn't pay for it: the studio producing his film did. In one social media post he pointed out the absurdity of trying to look like a superstar when, unlike you or I, they don't do it alone.

Some of our motivations for health now also come from people who we're led to believe are just like us. On social media, we're trained to think that normal everyday people take photos with their smartphones of their perfect bodies, so this is seen to be an attainable ideal for us. Yet, some research suggests that over half of women edit and alter their social media posts. That also doesn't take into account the dozens or more photos they take until they get the most flattering one. Social media is as unreal as mainstream media.

Not only are these external messages unhelpful, they're contrived. How motivating is it to chase an ideal that is completely unrealistic or manufactured? It might get us moving for a little while, or eating well for some time, but in the long run this lack of realistic expectation just makes everything worse. It destroys our confidence along with our goals. And when this runs into low self-esteem or poor body image, we're even less likely to take up healthy behaviours. However, Professor Thøgersen-Ntoumani says that, although we might start out our health journey like this, it is possible to cultivate true, internal and fulfilling motivation that is sustainable for our health.

One of the other ways our motivation can be upset is by the feelings of guilt that accompany failure. I told Professor Thøgersen-Ntoumani that I had felt an immense amount of guilt for not going running that morning. As expected, guilt is not a great motivator because it lacks an important aspect that is good for our mental and physical wellbeing. She reminded me of the value of self-compassion.

Self-compassion, or the ability to be kind to yourself if you miss a workout or eat something you told yourself you wouldn't, actually helps us to keep going in the long run. Self-compassion has been associated with the ability to sustain healthy behaviours, as well as have better body image, which might in turn help us show up and engage in those things we're trying to do for our health. A lack of self-compassion leads us to disordered eating, including eating disorders, binge eating or not having enough nutritional food. Self-compassion, a sense of kindness when we falter and a willingness to dust ourselves off and try again, may well be an important factor in our health that we can all learn.

Since health is something we value and recognise the importance of, I have wondered why health is not motivation enough? Some estimates say that by following a healthful diet, doing physical activity, limiting alcohol and stress, and not smoking, we extend our lives by 11–14 years. And those years are good, too, with less chronic disease to contend with. Why is this not enough?

I have to confess that when I meet someone through my work who is not meeting these targets, I try to reason that I want them to quit smoking or exercise more because 'it's good for them'. And it is; we know it is on so many fronts. And yet, we can't quite make that leap between knowing that's how we become healthy and actually doing those things. Where is the hold up?

First of all, we're starting with the big assumption that all people want to be healthier. Yet, that isn't always true. Some research suggests that less than 10 per cent of smokers want to quit and 30 per cent of people aren't interested in exercise. Studies in the US show that just 2.7 per cent of Americans meet targets for healthy living. They're not lofty goals either; they are eating nutritious foods, being active, maintaining a healthy body-fat level and not smoking. These appear pretty straightforward.

From all of the research I've read, and the experts I have spoken to, the reasons are vast. Look at your own reasons for skipping a workout or eating something you've told yourself you wouldn't. It can be hard. Life gets in the way of your workout and many of us are time-poor these days. Some days we're exhausted or perhaps the gym is too expensive. Healthy food can take time to prepare and it's easier to order in. Maybe you think illness won't happen to you or, if it does, it's years in the future and medicine will be able to fix it by then. Sometimes you just say 'screw it' and bite into something you know is unhealthy anyway.

Most of us understand what we need to do to be healthy and, on some level, we understand how important that is. But we have lost sight along the way as individuals and as a society. The result is a growing number of people who are dealing with everything from low self-esteem to disordered thinking, restrictive eating and strict exercise patterns, to full-blown preventable disease.

We all think that because we're free beings we have the bulk of control in our own hands. We choose what to eat, we choose whether or not to smoke, to drink or to sleep in or get up and exercise instead. And this is a message that we're fed daily: that you just need to want it more, to use your willpower to overcome your dangerous and self-indulgent habits. Instagram models show us pictures of before and after their self-realisation that they were once 'fat, unhappy party girls' and now they have 'banging bodies' (real quote from an Instagram health coach). All you need to do to share in this happiness and beauty is sign up to their program. You just need to want it and it's yours.

That's simply not the full picture. Despite the fact that virtually all of us have the freedom to choose our workout or our meals, this happens in an environment where our choices are guided by advertising, policy, our peers' opinions and the messages we've internalised over the years. If change were easy, everyone would do it. Every day, I see how people are not able to change what they need to for the sake of their health. Just think of all those unused gym memberships. We're buying into the surface markers but not progressing past that point.

We seem to think that by providing motivation in the form of knowledge, aspirational images or sometimes shame we can turn the tide. We've been doing that for some time now and, guess what, things are getting worse not better.

Wellness – it's not for everyone

The other point to make here is that living a healthy lifestyle has plenty of barriers to it. There are dozens of reasons why someone might not be able to eat well or exercise regularly. Healthy food is more expensive than less healthy alternatives and takes a bit of skill and time to prepare. Trust me, I'm not the world's greatest cook! Take away or pre-prepared food, which can be low in nutritional value, doesn't require much preparation, and tends to keep longer, which may make it cheaper. Some people simply cannot afford the gym but getting outside to walk or run, while cheap in comparison, requires a safe environment. Stress in our lives means that we're less likely to do the things we know are good for us. And, of course, for those who don't already fit the ideal body type or shape, their internalised stigma, as well as the discrimination faced from other people, has an impact on their ability to be healthy.

We're told what the 'healthiest' diet or best exercises are by a growing health and wellness industry that sets a standard for what being healthy actually is. Except there are two very obvious problems with this. Firstly, as I've mentioned, none of this is a real or reliable indicator of what health is. The second problem is that the wellness industry is expensive.

Keeping up with standards of health and wellness is not attainable for everyone, whether they're realistic or not. Buying wellness or health, even if it's just the outside shell not actual health, is the new lifestyle we aspire to. It's the new designer handbag, except that now, we're buying supplements and designer activewear. The wellness industry is really only available to people with high incomes. Health is off limits for a lot of people who don't make much money. Even buying fresh vegetables can be a stretch for those on lower incomes.

Since the vast proportion of the population cannot afford or cannot access all the wellness that is marketed to us, or sometimes even the most basic things that contribute to health, is it any wonder that so many of us remain unhealthy? And why have we allowed the wellness industry to get away with putting profit ahead of good-quality science, responsible communication and respect for the whole community? This is what is going on in an industry that is all about the money with very little regard for how its message is conveyed, and even if the message is accurate or good for us.

Even for those of us who have access to the aspirational wellness lifestyle that we're being sold, the outcomes are bound to be suboptimal. Since a large proportion of it doesn't work, is expensive or could be counter-productive in the long run, is it any wonder that our love affair with wellness isn't translating to real world health outcomes?

A new approach is urgently needed. An approach that doesn't hinge on beautiful bodies to inspire or a plethora of gyms and diets to choose from. An approach that is based in science not marketing. A way that shows compassion, rather than seeking to embarrass and belittle. A way that embraces our physical, mental, emotional and social health over simplistic or superficial motivations.

There are barriers at every turn stopping us from being healthy: copious amounts of advertising for foods that are not nutritious, the cost of healthy eating, finding time to exercise, finding a safe place to exercise, the cost of participating in sport and many more. These are all things that need to be addressed to give us a path without constant resistance to engage in health.

One thing that needs to change is *how* we're telling people to be healthy. A multi-billion-dollar industry has been built around this promise. Except that it doesn't have very much to do with health. Marketed as magic pills or quick fixes with young and beautiful people showing us what is possible, what a beautiful and happy body looks like, we're told that these external, superficial markers are the only way to measure and achieve success.

We all have to learn what it is to be healthy and one important way to do this is by unhooking this concept of healthy equalling beauty. Because it does not. Using beauty as a surrogate for health or as a motivator for healthy behaviours is doing nothing but leading us down an unhelpful pathway. We should all be angry at the messages we have been sold. The idea that beauty is what we are striving for has been pushed as a way to serve many other purposes, none of which are in our individual or our collective best interests.

Think back to that definition of health: its vastness, with health encompassing so many facets of who we are and what we do. It's our physical health, which is not measured by weight alone or by the attractiveness of our bodies. Physical health has many different parts to it, some of which we're still learning to measure or achieve. The so-called attractive or unattractive exterior of a body is not enough to be called healthy or unhealthy.

Not occurring in isolation, health also means we're mentally or emotionally healthy. It means that we're happy and fulfilled in the various parts of our lives. This means we have reasonable self-esteem and a healthy respect and pride in what our bodies and minds can do. It means that we have healthy relationships with other people, with food and exercise and with the world around us. It does not mean constant punishment by way of exercise or diet or restriction.

The different aspects of health do not happen independently of each other, and health is not cultivated away from the strengths and weaknesses of society. Health is contingent on the way the world around us is made and functions. We need to live in a world that supports us in these goals and doesn't prioritise profit and taking advantage of people's desire to be beautiful or attractive.

The ultimate goal here is to shift our focus from the things we currently use to denote healthy. To shift our focus away from gym memberships, activewear and diets, and to cut out our desperate need to engage with an entire industry designed to sell us health but really just feeding the insecurities and maladaptive habits that are actually making us sicker and poorer. Our reliance on this industry and our obsession with beautiful bodies in social media and magazines only serves industry, it doesn't serve our best interests.

The fitness, diet and wellness industries don't really pay attention to the science of health. They live by a different set of principles and that is to suck us in. At best, they are simply ignorant of what they do and how it's not helpful. For the majority of us, these industries continue to feed into the many barriers that actually stop us from being healthy.

To live a healthy life, we are going to have to change things radically. We need to change policy and learn new science, which is no small task. We need to learn to motivate ourselves and each other to be healthy in ways that are sustainable, by making us look to ourselves and our own lives and engage on a deeper level than attractiveness or beauty. We need to develop the skills to live a life that is truly healthy and goes far beyond the superficial.

That is why what we're doing isn't working. It's because it's not designed to. It's high time we worked out what will.

Chapter 3

DIET IS A FOUR-LETTER WORD

'Don't listen to your inner fatty.
She's an evil bitch who wants bread.'

UNKNOWN

I can pinpoint the exact moment in my life when my healthy relationship with food was damaged. Prior to this, I ate what I wanted (and needed) and really didn't have many problems with it. When I was a young medical student, I joined a gym and was approached by one of the personal trainers who thought I might do well in body building. I loved a challenge and enjoyed the gym at that stage, so embraced the task with gusto. Had I known what I know now, I would have rejected virtually everything he had to say. My training was not just about lifting weights and staying fit: a large part of it was an incredibly restrictive diet.

I still bear the scars of this time and know the prescription off by heart. A third of a cup of oats and two egg whites for breakfast, followed by a mid-morning protein shake. Lunch was half a cup of brown rice, vegetables and lean protein. Preferably tuna, which, to be honest, I hated. The only respite for the day was the mid-afternoon fruit snack (but no bananas or berries or melon). Dinner was a few hundred grams of meat with only green veggies. Bedtime was hunger. Actually, all day, every day was hunger.

I lost an enormous amount of weight. I also lost the will to live. I was grumpy and thin and wildly anti-social as I travelled everywhere with my protein shaker and plastic containers barely half-filled with food. My mum was rightly worried about the thin air I was consuming and would encourage a cheeky bowl of ice cream here and there. After she went to bed, I would finish the whole tub because I was so deprived during the day. Eventually, I caved and quit this stupid quest; the nail in the coffin was breaking my wrist at netball, the resulting x-ray showing that I had osteopenia, thinning of my bones. It's quite likely that it was caused by losing too much weight too quickly. I saw a dietitian afterwards who was furious about the dreadful advice I had been given and tried to steer me back to normality.

This experience had shown me how to develop an eating disorder and provide my body with completely inadequate nutrition. It amazes me that I had enough food and nutrients to be able to go to medical school at that stage, let alone train twice a day. I am still angry about that period in my life; angry with myself for being so vulnerable to the lure of a challenge and for not being more sceptical of the utter garbage I was buying into. I'm unhappy with myself mainly because from that moment on my relationship with food was incredibly damaged. I'm also furious that someone hid behind a qualification; a flimsy one at that. It infuriates me that a random personal trainer at the gym thought for a moment that he knew enough about nutrition to give out advice that was nothing short of harmful. What should have clued me in to his lack of smarts was the time he explained the physics of exercise to me. 'It is just like Albert Einstein said, every action has an equal and opposite reaction.' If you don't know basic science, you shouldn't be talking about it, mate.

The world of diets and eating programs is a deep, dark dive into some behaviours that are questionable and advice that is at best stupid and at worst dangerous. So many Facebook groups and diet books publish food advice that demonises sugar, fruit and certain vegetables. I found a diet that counts macros (macronutrients – carbohydrates, fats and protein) in all foods and demands that every ounce of food be weighed before and after cooking to allow accurate calculation. The same diet also encourages its followers to take a set of kitchen scales to a restaurant and weigh the food when eating out.

One diet, created by a popular Beverly Hills plastic surgeon, is not only unscientific, but each phase is named after a goal such as 'having a summer body', 'being red carpet ready' or simply, 'being hot'. There's an endless list of foods deemed to be the secret to health, such as alkaline water; even humble vegetables like cauliflower have gone from enhancing your mum's roast to being able to fight cancer better than chemotherapy. These diets prey on our desire to be attractive and slim; they make no mention of health, or rely on flimsy interpretations of science. In fact, they often disregard sound nutrition science. Many encourage a zealous following of one self-described expert's mantra while simultaneously promoting distrust in medical professionals and science.

Popular diets or eating plans come under fire by nutrition professionals for being fads. They often communicate contradictory dietary advice that differs from accepted science, with some promoting dangerous exclusion of whole food groups that have real health benefits. An Australian study of the dietary advice promoted online showed that when stacked against current dietary guidelines, most of the six online diets they examined that were promoted by celebrities or other unqualified people were nutritionally unsound. Some of these diets promoted overly restrictive eating or declared groups of food as unhealthy, despite evidence to the contrary. Between them, these people and their social media accounts had millions of followers who were exposed to faulty food advice.

The knowledge of people telling us what to eat ranges from expert-level down to straight-up ignorant. A survey by LiveLighter in Australia showed that 44 per cent of people use the internet to access nutritional information and 12 per cent of people surveyed look to social media influencers for advice. Even fitness professionals such as personal trainers fail to understand proper nutrition. An Australian study of the expertise of personal trainers showed that their knowledge is limited, suggesting they shouldn't be dolling out food advice. Australian personal trainers study a minimum of 12 hours of nutrition science in the most basic course of study for accreditation. This is not nearly enough. Nutrition is a vital and complex subject, and yet it seems anyone with an Instagram account or a job in a gym is telling us how to lose weight, be beautiful and healthy; it's causing untold damage.

There is no doubt that nutrition is important to health. Food is also central to our culture and how we interact and socialise with each other. Food even has a role to play in the health of our planet. So why are we so intent on listening to people or corporations who do not have our best interests at heart? Food is vital and yet we're willing to learn about it from anyone who says they know something. In my job, it would be the equivalent of having your heart surgery performed by someone with a social media account who Googled how to do it. We wouldn't accept that, yet that's pretty much what we do every day when it comes to advice about health and food. I'm not a dietitian or a nutritionist but I do believe in science and I understand the importance of what we eat to health and disease. And I am sick and tired of the way we are all being misled and even damaged in relation to food.

We are what we eat

Most of us seem to have a basic level of understanding that what we eat is important to our health and wellbeing. However, it's not easy for a lot of people to understand the finer details of a healthy diet. An American study demonstrated that nearly half of the people surveyed thought it was easier to do their taxes than it was to eat healthily. While we may think we know what is healthy, when we're pressed for the details of nutritious food and a balanced diet, they elude us.

It's essential that we know exactly what healthy foods and a nourishing diet looks like. How much we know about nutrition seems to correlate with how well we eat. In a US study of 1351 people, having a good knowledge of nutrition was directly linked to eating a healthier diet. Most Americans erroneously think that carbohydrates, sugar and fat are the main culprits in weight gain when, in fact, all macronutrients have the power to adversely affect our health if we eat too much of them.

Knowledge is power but when it comes to nutrition we haven't got the knowledge – so we definitely lack the power.

One of the earliest reasons that scientists and doctors started investigating the role of what we eat was the rise in heart disease. These early studies found that diet is key; initial research singled out fat as the biggest culprit. Groups of people eating a Mediterranean diet were studied and found to be leading long, happy, healthy lives. This influenced the first US dietary guidelines, published in 1977, which recommended a low-fat diet and blamed eggs for high cholesterol and heart disease. These early scientific studies on which the US guidelines were based have subsequently been re-examined, leading to the dietary advice being revised. Eggs, nuts and olive oil, once demonised, have now been found to be healthy and returned to the lists of recommended food. Many Western countries followed similar dietary guidelines, advocating fruit, vegetables, complex carbohydrates and limited amounts of sugar and fats, sometimes using a pyramid symbol to explain the relative proportions. The public was told: this is what's good for you. No further explanation was forthcoming. I do wonder how much this paternalistic attitude has contributed to our distrust in guidelines.

When we talk about the power of nutrition in health, what we're often discussing is disease-prevention. A large study published in the *Journal of the American Medical Association* looked at the dietary patterns of those people in the US who had died of heart disease, stroke or diabetes in one year. In the study, 45 per cent of the deaths, a total of 318,656, were found to be diet-related. It's important to note that there are a number of complex factors involved in analysing health and disease. However, this kind of research does point to why we need to be concerned with food. People who eat well, exercise, avoid smoking and maintain a healthy body weight halve their risk of heart disease and lead a longer life. WHO dietary guidelines limit the intake of saturated fats and trans fats and encourage eating fruits, vegetables, legumes, nuts and grains, which are thought to increase life expectancy. In addition, a diet high in fibre slashes your risk of heart disease by 40–50 per cent. These are big and important factors in living a long, healthy life.

Diet is also promoted as vital to weight loss. After some research studies concluded that you couldn't outrun a bad diet, social media stars and bloggers started to focus on this. Research has shown that if we compare the contribution of diet and exercise to weight loss, diet is more important – we lose more body fat if we reduce what we eat. However, health is not just diet-related and exercise is very good at reducing the amount of fat that sits around our organs – which is what actually causes disease. While the bloggers may be right that a good diet is vital to weight loss, they are simplifying things. Weight loss is partly about diet and exercise, but also about where you live, how much money you earn and your genetics. Kale isn't going to make you wealthy or move you to a higher socio-economic area and these factors are really big players in health and disease. That being said, because around 20 per cent of people who are deemed skinny or normal weight are still at risk for illness from lifestyle factors, everyone, regardless of their weight, needs to be eating a healthy diet. And we must make that available to everyone, not just people who can afford a daily Instagram-worthy smoothie bowl. Everyone deserves the health benefit of good food.

One of the problems I see with this method of communicating

Is food medicine?

No, it really isn't. Medicine is medicine. Food and our dietary patterns (what we eat over a period of time) can impact whether or not we develop disease. But to say that every bite that you take is making you sicker or healthier oversimplifies nutrition and devalues medicine. We're living in a time when science and medicine are devalued; the practice of Western medicine has been so unsatisfactory for so many patients that it's understandable people want some autonomy back. Food may form an integral part of disease management but save for a handful of medical conditions (coeliac disease springs to mind), it doesn't cure anything.

the importance of disease prevention is that it's inherently negative. We don't feel we're adding something of value to our lives because a lifetime of disease seems so far away when we're young. Or perhaps we get this sense that it will never happen to us, or that we'll do something about that disease *if* it happens. Or just take a pill. Prevention is infinitely better than anything I can do as a surgeon, for example. Research is showing that our lifestyle diseases are not only cutting our lives short, they are also leaving us living with higher amounts of debilitating, chronic disease. In science, the value of nutrition is often communicated in terms of avoiding disease but on social media the focus is more diffuse. Good food is promoted for beauty, thinness, clear skin and better sleep, with perhaps a vague mention of health.

At the same time, most of the benefits of diet are talked about in the media as ways to lose weight and, of course, being thinner is commonly seen as more attractive. We equate this slim, beautiful figure with being healthier, but that is wrong. Because we are so keen to lose weight to look a certain way, we miss out on the important part played by food in preventing disease and making us well. Helping to maintain a healthy body weight is just one way food can keep us healthy. Food can also influence everything from how our cells work to the bacteria that live in our gut. What we ought to be talking about is good health equating to a longer, happier life, free of disease. Or the ability to fuel our bodies to do the tasks we need or want to do. Focusing on weight and beauty just means we only eat to make our body *look* a certain way, not to make our lives better.

For years, people have wanted the vast body of nutritional knowledge in the form of simple pieces of advice. Bloggers and social media influencers take advantage of this to promote the benefits of a particular food or food element. We're told a single component such as an antioxidant in a blueberry leads to a single physical response such as clear skin or gut health. We're obsessing over details and completely losing sight of the bigger picture. And the bigger picture is that we eat food, not nutrients. This reductionist approach and focus on minutiae adds to the confusion around nutrition. While we know more than ever, if we can't communicate clearly this will never translate to better dietary choices.

Why we eat what we do

The push to eat well tries to focus on health and avoiding disease. It's hard to understand why people who know that healthy food is good for them can't quite commit to eating it full-time. Which means that knowing how to be healthy actually isn't enough when it comes to what we eat. Far from what popular opinion tell us, what we eat has only a little to do with willpower, and a lot to do with everything from taste to biology to what we can afford.

Hunger is obviously the most important reason for eating. Our bodies need food, they need the macronutrients (protein, fat and carbohydrates) and they need the micronutrients such as vitamins and minerals for the body to function the way it's supposed to. Hunger cues, such as a rumbling stomach, let us know we need to eat and then we feel full and satisfied afterwards. Whether or not we feel satiated depends on many factors, including how much we eat. Protein makes us feel the most satisfied, followed by carbohydrates and finally fat. The energy density of the food is important with high-energy density meals or foods sometimes leaving us wanting more. This hunger-satiety biological drive is fundamental but can be shifted and damaged by all of the other cues around us.

If it were as simple as relieving hunger, the challenge of eating well would be dead easy to overcome. Biology has also given us the desire for palatable, tasty food. Over our lifetime we develop a preference for the foods that taste good to us or provide comfort and joy. It's the palatability and enjoyment of sugary, fatty foods that causes us to accidentally overconsume them. Research has shown that if we enjoy a food, we tend to reach for it spontaneously. This is not an inherently bad thing, but if those foods are easy to access, it becomes easy to overeat calorie-dense food.

Another issue is cost, and how we have been taught to choose and prepare foods. Many studies have shown a link between poverty and lower consumption of fruit and vegetables. US research has shown that people like the convenience of fast food but are also attracted to an outlet with a children's playground. Another study looked at young people at a music festival; even those who planned to buy healthy food ended up buying unhealthy food due to lack of nutritionally sound choices. In the context of our food preferences, criticising people for not eating well is extremely hypocritical. We allow food outlets to take advantage of all the things that make us overeat, such as taste, availability and low price, and then blame people for laziness or lack of willpower, when the sheer market force of cheap unhealthy food makes it difficult to create a culture around healthier alternatives.

It's no wonder that we see poor nutrition contributing to disease. Despite the fact that we know more than ever about how food keeps us well, translating that knowledge from scientists and nutritionists to the public is challenging. The overwhelming message is that exerting willpower and discipline over what you eat is the easiest thing in the world. It's a message I've heard colleagues tell patients for years, with a focus on that person's weight and appearance rather than their wellbeing. This creates an opportunity for the diet industry to swoop in and make things, at times, a whole lot worse.

Do diets even work?

When we talk about a 'diet', there are two definitions. The first is a scientific definition that covers the pattern of foods that someone eats. The second is the one we're probably more familiar with, that is a multi-billion-dollar, controversial industry. In it, a diet is a supervised and regulated pattern of eating that is done to lose weight or manage a disease. Diets are commonly the topic of best-selling books or chatter among friends or family where we're sold a quick and easy way to lose weight. Diets are so common that research studies have shown that 20 per cent of adults at any one time are on a diet. Those rates rise to above 60 per cent if we look at the number of young women on a diet and some studies have estimated that the average woman spends 17 years of her life on a diet. Dieting is so widespread that we think it's normal to restrict our food aggressively, when research would suggest that that is a convenient and a potentially dangerous lie we've bought into.

When I think of spending 17 years of my life watching every morsel I consume, I really want to know why we do this, because it seems like a big fat waste of time. The two main reasons people give for dieting is to lose weight and to be healthy. Research has shown that around half of those dieting do so for health reasons, but around a third do so to look better. Motivation is very important; a large body of research has shown that, for women in particular, dieting to look better is problematic. A Canadian study that looked at motivation found that women who diet for external reasons such as appearance were more likely to diet in an unhealthy fashion, severely restricting what and how much they eat. An Australian study of women dieters found a worrying association between dieting and appearance, including a tendency to be attracted to diets promoting quick and easy solutions.

While we may like to think that we're mainly dieting to be healthier, research doesn't support this. Cultural influences are a big factor and, for young women, very few of these are centred around health – they're about fashion and beauty. In addition, people sacrifice health for weight loss and associate health with a dress size. Some studies have suggested that while dieters say they want to be healthy, appearance may actually be the underlying goal. Again, we see associations with psychological distress and disordered eating, which is not the same as an eating disorder but rather a wide range of abnormal eating behaviours that include chronic restrained eating and bingeing, among others.

Ironically, if you're dieting for these external reasons, it's even less likely you will achieve your goal. A number of research articles have shown that if you focus on health by following good dietary guidelines, such as adding vegetables rather than eating less and being restrictive, your health improves, you lose weight and you're less likely to binge eat.

Anti-diet sentiment is growing all the time, both among scientists and the general public. Serious concerns have been raised about the way dieting fails to help you lose weight and contributes to binge eating. It is thought to be psychologically damaging because it promotes unhealthy body image and emotional trauma. Since most dieters either don't lose the weight or lose it and regain it, this makes them feel like a failure. Diet culture has promoted the idea that our bodies can be easily changed and shaped and that everyone who uses the right diet and exercise plan can achieve their goal. And that once you do, the rewards are enormous: health, happiness, attractiveness, fame and respect. This kind of drivel is perpetuated by genetically gifted Instagram models and couldn't be further from the truth.

Every day someone tells us about a miracle diet. Unlike every other diet you've ever heard of, this one will really work. It is scientifically sound and has helped Bev from Brisbane (Bristol or

Boston) lose those stubborn baby kilos. Or helped Darren get rid of his dad bod. The truth is that no single diet has been shown to be better than any other diet. Restricting in any fashion to achieve a calorie deficit will result in at least temporary weight loss; it's not magic. Science shows that the majority of dieters experience weight loss initially but regain it over time. Anyone promising a miracle breakthrough is lying or grossly misrepresenting what we know.

Aside from the psychological fallout, we now know the futility of dieting. One of the most public displays of weight loss happens in reality TV show *The Biggest Loser*. Researchers from the US followed 16 contestants from the show who had successfully lost, on average, 58 kg each. They put the participants through specialised laboratory tests to measure their metabolic rate and body composition and also watched what they ate and how they exercised. All the competitors, bar one, regained the weight. Researchers also found that their metabolic rate slowed as they lost weight, which made sustained weight loss hard. In addition, the aggressive way in which contestants dieted and exercised was completely unsustainable in the real world. The reality is that for the TV contestants, just reducing their energy by 20 per cent would have kept them on the right track, but their overly strict regimen doomed them to failure.

Another meta-analysis of popular, commercially available diets showed that at least 30 per cent of people don't complete the diet and, in addition to that, some plans result in a weight loss of less than 5 per cent of body weight. A number of research studies have actually shown that a lot of dieters end up gaining back all the weight they've lost, plus more. Diets promise you the world but deliver absolutely nothing.

By highlighting the science behind the struggle, *The Biggest Loser* research hit a nerve with the public who then saw how difficult weight loss can be. Our bodies do not like losing weight; if they are forced to they undergo a number of changes that actually encourage weight gain. Our bodies are smart: they have an infinite network of hormones and cell processes that maintain everything about us in such tight control that it's hard to measure. This process is called homeostasis and it's unconscious and immutable. It is so vital to our wellbeing that disrupting it leads to disease.

Homeostasis is responsible for keeping our weight in a certain range; some experts suggest that we have a predetermined 'set point' for our weight that is bloody hard to shift. Our weight is controlled by several regions in the brain, namely the cerebral cortex, limbic system and hypothalamus. The cerebral cortex is the outer most part of our brain, responsible for a lot of the higher functions, like decision making. The limbic system is important in emotions and their regulation. Hormones interact between the hypothalamus and our peripheral organs, such as the gut, pancreas, liver, muscle and fat, and these fall into two groups: those that increase our appetite and those that decrease it. Hormones or other signalling substances, such as neuropeptide Y, gastroinhibitory peptide and ghrelin, stimulate appetite. Others, such as proopiomelanocortin, leptin, cholecystokinin and insulin, suppress appetite. (Insulin is interesting in that it works in the brain to reduce appetite but when it's given to diabetics via injection it promotes weight gain.) External factors can affect this, such as saturated fat, which is thought to cause inflammation in the hypothalamus that can actually increase appetite signals. Although this system exists solely to make sure our bodies have enough to eat, it seems to lack the power to overcome tasty food, advertising or the complex psychology that surrounds our choice to eat more than we need. When we lose weight, the balance between these hormones is tipped in favour of stimulating appetite and seems to stay that way for quite some time.

It's not just our bodies that fight against weight loss; anyone who has ever been on a diet understands how temptation seems to be all around. Our environment promotes high-energy dense foods, large portion sizes and inactivity. We tend to think of giving in to this temptation as giving up or failing, but the world is set up to make us eat more and do less. So while we think that falling off the diet bandwagon is a personal failure, it's actually a combination of our body's normal hormonal response to weight loss, and a carefully constructed campaign in society to get us eating food and gaining weight.

Diets are not benign. If I were recommending surgery that had the same failure rate and far-reaching side effects and that also fought against the body's natural inclinations, nobody in their right mind would let me operate. And nor should they: the risks of dieting seem to outweigh the benefits. For the majority of people, diets don't work and they leave a trail of destruction. That's not to say that we should eat whatever is put in front of us. Our health is too precious for us not to pay attention to the role of nutrition. But the idea that we can simply use the latest and most successful diet to lose weight and be rewarded with good health, beauty and success is just too much of a false promise.

The diets we are being sold have been around for centuries and they still aren't the solutions we're looking for. Just like fashion, they cycle in and out of popularity as the human race looks for happiness and the cure for everything from disease to bigger bodies. Science is trying to unravel what works, what is best for certain people and how to make sure that the weight loss sticks. It's even far too early to call sugar or fat the sole reason why people are bigger; this also oversimplifies the science at hand. In the meantime, we continue to torture ourselves with diets that are largely destined to fail.

Paleo-keto-detox-clean-fasting: nutribollocks

For the best part of a century, diet fads have come and gone. In 1963 Weight Watchers was created, paving the way for a long list of diets such as the Cabbage Soup diet, Atkins, South Beach Diet and even Oprah Winfrey's Optifast, on which she's rumoured to have consumed just 400 calories per day for months. Now that diets are falling out of favour, this gap in the market is being filled with what I can only call a wolf in sheep's clothing. Rather than focusing on a limited diet with say a 12-week meal plan, what we have instead is a growth in tribes of nutritional ideology. They claim to be healthy habits or ways to live but they're just diets dressed up as healthy lifestyles.

Modern-day nutritional advice is doled out in the form of eating patterns such as Paleo, ketogenic, detox diets, clean eating and intermittent fasting. Clean eating has been gaining popularity in recent years with some surveys showing it as the most popular diet for under 25s in the US. A number of these diet plans are championed by celebrities, such as the Paleo diet, popularised by Australian chef Pete Evans and much loved at CrossFit gyms.

Celebrity American plastic surgeon Dr Terry Dubrow and his wife, Heather, who is a cast member on *Real Housewives of Beverly Hills*, are putting their spin on the ketogenic diet with their book, *The Dubrow Diet.*

The American Dietetic Association defines a fad diet as one that contains illogical information and distorted beliefs about food. This includes advertising that certain foods can cure disease or bring specific health benefits, including offering quick weight loss. For example, the Paleo diet claims to prolong life, enchance gut health, give you clear skin, promote better absorption of nutrients from food and also lead to sustained weight loss. Like most of these new-look diets, the claims are generally unsubstantiated. The Paleo diet is said to have evolved from the one followed by our paleolithic ancestors (who rarely lived past middle age); anthropologists have shown this to be historically inaccurate. From a nutritional standpoint, the Paleo diet cuts out important foods such as grains, which reduce the risk of bowel cancer and heart disease. A recent Australian study even asked whether Paleo might increase the risk of heart disease. A lack of wholegrains has been shown to increase the blood levels of a substance called trimethylamine-n-oxide (TMAO) which, when its levels are high, is associated with disease of the heart.

In addition, foods marketed as 'clean', 'guilt-free' or high in so-called miracle nutrients such as protein or vitamins and minerals are enjoying a surge in popularity, along with 'superfoods', which are marketed as the key to health and wellbeing. Despite the fact that the science behind these claims is either missing or grossly overstated, people are spending more and more money on these supposed elixirs. Social media is littered with these claims, including ones by Anthony William, a medium who uses his alleged gift to bring health to the masses. William maintains that celery juice can heal your liver, which flies in the face of all science.

A total of 60 per cent of shoppers in one US survey said they were trying to eat more protein for its health benefits. Sales of dietary supplements amounted to more than $US 41.2 billion last year, despite the fact that science says they do not work. Conversely, some foods, such as sugar, are being demonised as the root of all disease. Australian journalist Sarah Wilson, founder of the popular *I Quit Sugar* program, claimed that she managed her anxiety and depression by cutting out sugar, including the natural sugar from fruit, a statement that has no scientific support.

The fact remains that there is not enough good science to support following these diets; at best they are a loose interpretation of science. While each of these dietary approaches or nutritional obsessions can be challenged individually, there are broader issues at play. In the first instance, a large amount of this advice is completely unsupported by science and at times can even lead to harm. The indiscriminate cutting out of foods with nutritional value such as some fruits or vegetables and grains means that people are not deriving the important health benefits these foods bring. Foods that are purported to be 'super' or special are often significantly more expensive than regular foods of the same nutritional value, meaning that we could be wasting vast amounts of money. Clean eating and all of its cousins are generally pastimes of the upwardly mobile, given the requirements for unusual and pricey miracle ingredients and special kitchen tools.

These diets are supported by zealots who claim that, somewhere on the planet, a group of fisherman have eaten this way for centuries and haven't grown fat or had heart attacks. This appears to be backed by science but in reality, promoters of certain foods or diets take a slither of science (or bad science) and turn it into a crusade. Take the 'superiority' of low-carbohydrate diets. Low-carb proponents will point to some tiny scientific study that has major holes in its results and should not be relied upon, to prove their point of view is right. But it is an overstatement of authority and evidence. If you say 'research shows' with enough confidence, people tend to believe you. Dig deeper though and the science doesn't hold up or doesn't exist.

The certainty with which these diet proponents believe that they are doing a superior job of living adds yet another moral judgement. For example, telling people that they need to eat 'clean' judges those people who are not doing so as playing fast and loose with their health. After a news outlet said that the UK had reached 'peak lazy' for not making Instagram-worthy foods from scratch, dietitians Rosie Saunt and Helen West of The Rooted Project wrote an article for the *Huffington Post*, hitting back:

'Although this food-snob mentality may make people feel better about their own choices, it's really a judgemental attack on people's lives with no regard for their needs or circumstance. It's very easy for those sitting comfortably in the middle classes, knee deep in wellness and yoga pants, to turn up their noses at 'processed food' and declare it 'disgusting' and 'lazy'. Regardless of good intentions, or whatever our personal views about food, passing moral judgement on people's choices is never helpful.'

The growing distrust of the established science of nutrition and medicine means that when health-care professionals try to promote realistic messages or debunk bad science it provokes vicious outcries from the diet zealots. This boosts the idea that science is bad, people are being lied to and the diet-promoter is your saviour who has discovered the answers doctors have willingly hid from the public for years. The government-sponsored, scientifically based eating guidelines such as Eatwell in the UK and MyPlate in the US are sound. However, since they lack the miracle-cure status or sexiness of all those other diets, critics denounce them as outdated conspiracies to make us sick rather than well. Distrust makes breaking down these messages even harder still.

A backlash is now, gratifyingly, forming against what is termed nutribollocks. While there is no formal definition of nutribollocks, it's a way of describing foods and diets that are fads with the potential to harm people physically and psychologically. In the course of writing this book, following the blogs and social media accounts that perpetuate nutribollocks has been nothing short of soul-destroying. I've read the enormous amount of false information that hundreds of thousands of people are exposed to daily. The challenge comes in fighting this information. Dr Emma Beckett PhD, a nutritional researcher from the University of Newcastle, and Alan Flanagan, a nutrition postgraduate researcher at the University of Surrey, both acknowledge the noise of social media and the challenge that faces science communicators who are trying to get accurate and effective information out to the public. Both Beckett and Flanagan try to myth-bust some of the nonsense around nutribollocks in an effort to promote health over noise. Dietitians Saunt and West formed The Rooted Project with the specific intent of debunking false information and spreading good science.

The difficulty comes in weeding out the bad messages and hearing the good ones. We can be very trusting of someone who claims to have qualifications and on social media we tend to take seriously the opinions of someone who is attractive, famous or has a large following, regardless of whether their information is true or not. But verified accounts (the ones with the blue ticks) simply confirm the person's identity, not their expertise. It's a natural psychological phenomenon for people to overstate their ability. Research from *Harvard Business Review* shows that when total beginners learn a little bit about any topic, their confidence eclipses their accuracy. In other words, we back ourselves when we don't know nearly enough to do so. This is often called the Dunning–Kruger effect: confidence almost always outstrips knowledge when we don't have any to speak of.

When clean is too clean: orthorexia

'Clean eating' or any other dietary pattern can take over your life. If you've ever done this, or lived with someone who is following a strict plan, you'll know the lists of things you cannot possibly touch because you're eating clean, paleo or low-carb. It's taken me nearly 15 years to eat potatoes without berating myself for the enormous carb load. We have normalised this kind of behaviour so much that when we stop eating for a period of time we call it 'intermittent fasting' rather than a pathological behaviour.

In the 1990s, US doctor Steve Bratman coined the term 'orthorexia' to describe an extreme eating pattern undertaken for health reasons, which leads to malnutrition or impairment of daily functioning. It's not an eating disorder defined in the diagnostic manual for psychiatric disorders that strictly categorises other eating disorders. However, since the term was first described

20 years ago, research into the topic has grown with plenty of evidence supporting its existence.

Orthorexia is thought to start innocently with a choice to eat a healthy diet. Bratman, who was an alternative medical practitioner, prescribed such diets but soon noted that his patients were taking it too far. Dieting can become problematic when the diet is highly restrictive, obsessive and includes ideas of cleanliness, impurity and self-punishment for breaches. People with orthorexia don't lack interest in eating but are obsessed with food, which grows to become a bigger and bigger part of their life.

The clinical definition of orthorexia is still being worked out by researchers in this field. Nevertheless, the illness could be surprisingly common, depending on the group we look at. One study of Italians showed a prevalence of 6 per cent; another study of female Brazilian nutritionists found an alarming rate of 88.7 per cent. It's far too early to say how common this eating disorder is or even if it's becoming more prevalent.

However, as Instagram is full of posts on juice cleanses, meal supplements and fasting plans, we have to ask if our current obsession with image and the use of social media is contributing to this disorder. In a study of 680 social media users, researchers found that viewing Instagram correlated with orthorexic tendencies. This didn't apply to any other social media channel, probably because Instagram is the most image-based. It is also the social media feed with the highest number of followers – it's not uncommon to have tens of thousands – giving the Instagrammer a huge reach and a false air of authority.

Studies of personal trainers have found that they see extreme diet and exercise as completely legitimate health pursuits, despite evidence that they are harmful. Blogger and Instagram star Jordan Younger declared herself orthorexic in 2014 when, as 'The Blonde Vegan', she told tens of thousands of followers that she would stop giving out advice because she had suffered health problems as a consequence of her restrictive diet. These are the types of people who are reaching impressionable young women, fuelling problems around body image, weight, diet and exercise. Extreme dieting is not a legitimate pursuit, just as binge eating is harmful. The pendulum needs to swing to the middle, not the extremes.

Intuitive eating – the anti-diet answer?

One of the side effects of a century and a half of diet culture is that we have a huge and restrictive set of principles when it comes to food. We eat based on calories, or forbidden foods and hero foods with the aim of losing weight. Some of the emotions attached to food and diet are normal, such as liking a particular food or enjoying a birthday cake with your family. Others are not so helpful, such as crippling guilt over eating a piece of bread or a bar of chocolate.

Intuitive eating is almost an antithesis to dieting, letting us get back to understanding the cues and signals our bodies send us about eating. There is a set of 10 principles of intuitive eating: these involve rejecting diet culture, not labelling foods good, bad or forbidden, focusing on health rather than weight, and learning to understand when you're hungry and when you're full. It's a way of looking inwards for cues to eat, rather than outwards to models or diets or gym challenges. Tracy Tylka, a body image researcher and Professor of Psychology from Ohio State University, summarised intuitive eating around three basic principles: unconditional permission to eat, eating for physical rather than emotional reasons, and tuning into your body's cues for when it's hungry and when it's full. Chronic dieting is very good at cutting the ties we have with the needs of our bodies. For example, chronic dieting can actually disrupt the stomach's function, delaying the signals that get sent to your brain to say you're done. Before you know it, you've eaten way more than you needed to or intended to because your stomach has no idea what to do anymore.

Intuitive eating was first described by dieticians Evelyn Tribole and Elyse Resch as a way to eat for your body's need for food rather than for your emotions or the situation: 'A personal process of honouring health by listening and responding to the direct messages of the body in order to meet your physical and psychological needs.' Clinical nutritionist Laura Thomas PhD hailed it as a way to get off the chronic dieting merry-go-round.

Intuitive eating is finding its home in the fight for good health. Since its inception, it has spawned a number of research projects in areas including gut health, weight loss, polycystic ovarian syndrome and eating disorders. There is also some evidence to suggest that intuitive eating can improve our levels of good cholesterol (HDL) and lower bad cholesterol (LDL), which is great news for heart health.

The popularity of intuitive eating in the scientific community has shown some distinct benefits. It has been found to improve body satisfaction, improve the desire to exercise and improve self-compassion. In one study of 200 American university students, intuitive eating was also associated with having a lower BMI. However, intuitive eating is not a way to lose weight and dietitians

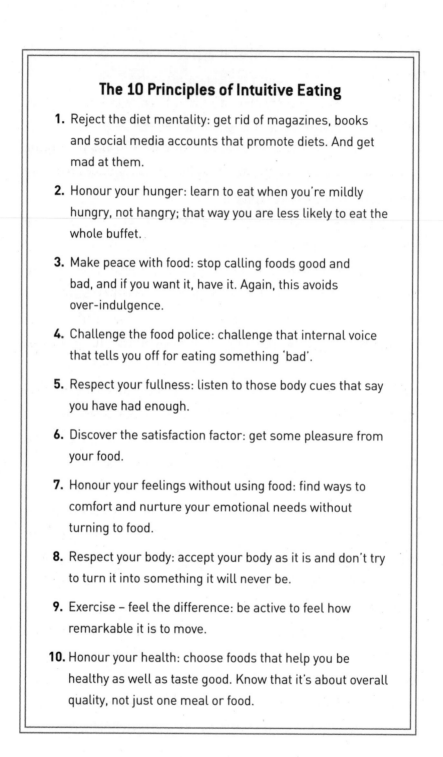

The 10 Principles of Intuitive Eating

1. Reject the diet mentality: get rid of magazines, books and social media accounts that promote diets. And get mad at them.

2. Honour your hunger: learn to eat when you're mildly hungry, not hangry; that way you are less likely to eat the whole buffet.

3. Make peace with food: stop calling foods good and bad, and if you want it, have it. Again, this avoids over-indulgence.

4. Challenge the food police: challenge that internal voice that tells you off for eating something 'bad'.

5. Respect your fullness: listen to those body cues that say you have had enough.

6. Discover the satisfaction factor: get some pleasure from your food.

7. Honour your feelings without using food: find ways to comfort and nurture your emotional needs without turning to food.

8. Respect your body: accept your body as it is and don't try to turn it into something it will never be.

9. Exercise – feel the difference: be active to feel how remarkable it is to move.

10. Honour your health: choose foods that help you be healthy as well as taste good. Know that it's about overall quality, not just one meal or food.

and nutritionists who practise in this area rightly caution people about this.

Intuitive eating is also not flexible eating, where people take smaller servings of food or compensate at the next meal if they overeat at one meal. Flexible eating still has elements of control, restriction and deprivation that feature in diets and does not have ties to physical or emotional health.

Intuitive eating sounds like a licence to eat whatever you want and Laura Thomas acknowledges that having a 'fuck it' day (or week) may happen, but this is a normal part of the process of your body learning what it needs. As she puts it, you might 'hang out in donut town for a couple of weeks, but it's not sustainable'. Ultimately, our bodies need good nutrition and good food because, when it boils down to it, we all want to feel well. We want energy and stamina and health. Research has demonstrated that intuitive eaters tend to have higher diet quality over all, which is really what we need for good emotional and physical health. It's not about denial or absolute freedom, but intuitive eating might be a holistic tool that has surprisingly good benefits on our health.

Those who promote intuitive eating as a weight-loss strategy come under heavy scrutiny from dietitians; it is not a weight-loss plan. However, avoiding the chronic yo-yo nature of dieting might in turn lead to weight loss or at least weight stabilisation. One study of overweight intuitive eaters pitted them against calorie counters: the calorie counters lost more weight. Some intuitive eaters lost weight, but not as much as the calorie counters. In general, intuitive eating isn't a way to lose weight and should never be considered a 'diet'. Just like dieters, intuitive eaters can slip back into old ways, losing their body awareness and internal cues.

Intuitive eating does need practice, just like any lifestyle change. It needs to come with education about good diet and exercise; it's not easy to abolish old habits and relearn what it means to be hungry, and we're doing it in a world that makes it a challenge. We're told to drink water if we're hungry, when really hunger necessitates food. We're served enormous portions that we finish, pushing past our feelings of fullness. Intuitive eating is vastly better than deprivation or stuffing yourself, and brings skills we desperately need but have forgotten. But it isn't a magic bullet; it's just one part of the solution when it comes to letting go of diets, diet culture and the havoc that they cause.

Chapter 4

BIKINI BODIES

'Would you rather be covered in sweat at the gym or covered in clothes at the beach?'

UNKNOWN

I grew up being active. Running, swimming, surfing and weight lifting were activities my whole family took part in – as an adult, these are my ways to keep fit, burn off steam and, if I'm honest, look and feel good. That does not mean that it comes easy; in fact, some days I absolutely despise working out and ignore my alarm. Other days, I get home after work and the last thing I feel like doing is going for a run. To stave off this tendency to skip a workout, I book into a gym class a couple of days a week.

One hot summer morning, I went to my gym for an hour-long circuit class of exercises designed to 'burn fat and tone long, lean muscles'; the sales pitch tapped into the trend to be lean and muscular. At the mid-point of the class, when a much-needed two-minute break was imminent, the perky instructor yelled out: 'Okay guys! We're gonna do 10 burpees and then plank for a minute in the break!' To me, a break is a break, not an opportunity for more torture. The class participants clearly had the same thought; the small group stared back at her, silently objecting by not moving. In true gym instructor fashion, she cheerily yelled commands. 'No? There is no no! Get planking!' So I half-heartedly stumbled my way through my burpees and plank, kissed my two-minute break goodbye and hoped she would melt away in the heat.

I felt like a child being yelled at to do their chores. I had come to this class of my own free will and yet, despite being an adult with autonomy, I was being made to feel like a naughty child, or a new army recruit, by a young woman in lycra. When did I agree to be barked at to do an exercise I hate, am not good at, at a time when I needed a nice water break and a moment to rest my tired muscles? I contemplated how this kind of forced activity could backfire by stopping people returning, because who wants to be yelled at on a Saturday morning? Breaks exist for a reason; to prevent injury and allow recovery. I thought about the dozens of trainers and class leaders I'd seen over the years, desperately trying to convince us by shouting that we did indeed want to feel close to death in order to get a decent workout. The military-style forced workout is so common it's on TV shows and in my local park, where a wall of a man is regularly seen yelling at a bunch of middle-aged mums to 'move their arses' up the hill. No wonder we hate exercise: it's being sold as punishment everywhere we look.

So many of these gyms and trainers sell the same formula. Hard work for a transformation; you get beaten up for eight weeks or more and have your fat measured and your weight documented in both numbers and pictures in various stages of undress. They trade in concepts like the 'new you' and 'guaranteed results' and swapping your free will when you walk in the door for the instruction of perky or tyrannical instructors. A US woman successfully sued a gym after a trainer turned up the resistance on her exercise bike so high that she became exhausted, fell off and broke her ankle. Exercise is now something not to be enjoyed but endured in the name of your ultimate goal and your future self, who will apparently thank you for the sore muscles in exchange for whittling away your waistline. It's a trend that was once the domain of popular TV shows and is now everywhere, as we sacrifice enjoyment in order to be better-looking versions of ourselves.

The Biggest Loser is one of the original transformation shows. In dozens of countries around the world, viewers tune in to watch men and women receive tough love from their trainers while talking about their 'journey' to becoming happier, fitter and smaller. They sweat through mud and humidity as trainers yell and scream at them to keep going despite their obvious exhaustion. From the comfort of our couches, we revel in watching them go through hell. In the show's finale, the newly slim – and therefore happy and healthy – contestants walk out on stage and are pictured next to their former selves. The 'old' self, as well as being bigger, is depicted as sad and lost. The new self? Well; they're a smiley, slimmer figure who often makes some sort of gesture to exorcise their old self from their life. We love that moment of transformation, to see just how far they've come from disgusting and sad bodies to slim, tanned and seemingly happy ones.

Selling transformations, summer bodies or ripped rigs in the form of exercise programs is booming business. There are countless programs offering the best exercises or regimens to take you from woe to wow, usually in a short time frame. They use what is touted as a never-before-seen combination of exercises designed to give you the waistline of your dreams. These programs often share the before-and-after pictures of people who have followed the daily exercise prescriptions and, just like on TV, they go from looking frumpy and sad to happy and beautiful. The programs are the latest iteration of diet and fitness culture and come with slogans like 'bikini body ready', 'summer bodies are made in the winter' and 'get shredded for summer'.

Kayla Itsines has built a large empire of followers who call themselves 'Kayla's Army'. The Adelaide personal trainer has the bank balance to match, being named in 2018 as Australia's richest person under 40, with an estimated net worth of $486 million. Considering she charges $20 a month to access her exercise app 'SWEAT', it's hardly surprising she's amassed a fortune. Itsines first rose to fame by selling the *Bikini Body Guide*, in which she claims that women around the world are making 'permanent and sustainable changes' to their lives by doing her workout three times a week. On her Instagram account, which has millions of followers, Itsines often posts pictures of women transformed by her program, using the same sad-bigger-before/happy-slim-after formula. Although her program is 12 weeks long, Itsines' success stories often show pictures of people who have used the program for much longer – even up to years down the track – to achieve remarkable 'overnight' results.

Kayla Itsines' followers are voracious consumers of stories of Kayla and her program. Her 27-minute circuit style workouts are supposed to be done in the comfort of your own home but often require a fair amount of equipment. Via the app, users are encouraged to share a 'sweaty selfie' to celebrate finishing their workout of burpees, squats and ab exercises. The hashtag #BBG, for Bikini Body Guide, has millions of pictures on Instagram, as does #DeathByKayla, which represents the gruelling nature of her workouts.

Itsines isn't alone in jumping on the body transformation bandwagon. In the UK, 'The Body Coach', Joe Wicks, has amassed an equally impressive following with his claims that he can make you *Lean in 15,* the title of his wildly successful book. Wicks studied to be a physical education teacher at university and, although he is a staunch advocate of good nutrition, he holds no formal nutritional qualification. His nutritional advice is often (correctly) criticised for his scientific-sounding but generally bullshit claims that calories don't matter if you have good fats. His recipes have even been compared to KFC in terms of their calorie content. Wicks also encourages cutting out some vegetables (yes, vegetables) because of their high carb content, particularly on days when you're working out so your workouts are 'carb-depleted'. Carbohydrates are an important fuel for active people, with research on athletes who consume low-carbohydrate diets showing a decline in their athletic performance: they simply lack the fuel their active body needs. This may actually be bad for our immune systems and can also encourage cortisol spikes, which can increase visceral fat deposition.

Wicks' Instagram account peddles the benefits of high-intensity interval training (HIIT), for just 15 minutes a day in your living room, to millions of followers. The workouts are complemented by his recipes, which are designed for a very active exercise program. Which seems to indicate that you're eating a butt-load of food and you need to burn it off. All of this information is available in his uber-bestselling books; like Itsines, Wicks uses transformational pictures of successful users of his program to sell his lifestyle. Did I also mention that he is a big fan of the 'no excuses' approach to health? It doesn't matter about money, gym memberships, parenting, working and so on, you just need to do it. I don't think I need to point out that this is unrealistic for many people. Joe's perky persona is raking in the big bucks with a 90-day program which is allegedly tailor-made for you, based on your weight, coming at a sweet £97 ($AU 150). But don't forget, he literally told you two minutes ago that you don't need to spend money to be healthy, unless, of course, it's going to him. Wicks promises 'real people, real results in real time' and it's plain to see that perceived authenticity is a vital part of his pitch. Don't get me wrong, Wicks seems like a nice bloke who wants people to exercise, which is great; however, his program has some holes in it that aren't plugged by science.

Of course, Wicks and Itsines aren't alone. Virtually everyone is sharing their transformation and a large number of people are making money out of it. Former Australian *The Biggest Loser* trainer Michelle Bridges sells programs for losing the last 5 kg of weight with an impressive collection of online courses, books, activewear and lunchboxes designed to replicate the tough-love approach she took on the TV program. Multiple celebrities, including *The Only Way Is Essex* cast members and pop stars, make workout videos showing you how to get their 'bikini bodies' by doing a series of exercises in your living room. *Men's Health* magazine frequently features a man who undergoes an eight-week transformation with the final prize being a cover photo and multiple-page spread in the popular magazine where he shows off his ripped physique. Cult gym phenomenon F45, where participants work out for 45 minutes in what's called a 'team training environment', run four eight-week challenges per year; the people with the biggest transformations (featuring photos in your undies with body fat percentages) win large cash prizes.

The lure of transforming an unhappy, round body to a slimline bikini body is hard to ignore; people everywhere spend money and time to achieve that through an exercise program which promises to deliver the world. There are endless numbers of people making a lot of money out of the fact that we want to look better. They promote their exercise programs as the answer to all of your body concerns, with health as a side effect. Although she has tried to distance herself a little from it, Kayla Itsines' program is still called a 'bikini body guide', not a way to be healthy.

It's hard to understand the motivation for these programs. Are we doing one-size-fits-all workouts for a stronger heart and healthy mind or are we doing it in the hopes of seeing the same mind-blowing transformations that are plastered all over Instagram? And if we are doing it for the abs or the pecs or whatever, is that really a bad thing? As with our diets, modern life is providing us with mixed messages about exercise and body image in a way that emphasises form over function and promises the world with variable delivery. And, just like all of the inconsistent information out there promising health, it's hard to know what is good for us and what isn't.

Extreme makeovers

Of course, if you don't want to spend time and money working on your bikini body, there is another way to transform yourself: cosmetic surgery and procedures. According to a report from the Australian College of Cosmetic Surgery, Australians spent

$AU 1 billion on cosmetic procedures in 2018, making us the country with the highest number of cosmetic procedures per capita in the world. Roughly 500,000 cosmetic procedures were carried out, including 20,000 breast enhancements, 30,000 liposuction procedures and $AU 350 million worth of Botox injections. A study into breast implants revealed an overall complication rate of 31.8 per cent following saline implants and 11.7 per cent following silicone implants, with revision surgery costing over $AU10 million a year.

The US has usually led the way in this area. A 2018 US survey reported that 18 million people had undergone surgical and minimally invasive cosmetic procedures in that year. The most popular were breast augmentation, followed by liposuction, nose reshaping, eyelid surgery and tummy tucks. The fastest growing procedure was vaginal rejuvenation, including labiaplasty, which increased by 23 per cent. The most popular non-surgical procedure continued to be injectables, with Botox coming in at number one. Of course, no-one likes to admit their bikini body might be the result of surgery rather than hard work, so you'd be hard-pressed to find any of those influencers admitting to going under the knife.

Plastic surgery makeovers as a road to the 'new you' have even featured on TV shows such as *Extreme Makeover* and *The Swan*. More recently, TV show *Botched* has provided a much more realistic look at the downside of plastic surgery. In this show, patients seek expert help to undo some of the horrific complications related to the pursuit of a perfect body part.

Plastic surgeons have been criticised for their heavy reliance on highly sexualised transformation pictures in their advertising. Professor Emerita Nichola Rumsey openly criticised this approach to plastic surgeons in 2018, stating that this reliance on 'soft porn' imagery contributed to body-image concerns and underplayed the seriousness of invasive surgery. Not all plastic surgery is bad, with the growth of procedures following major weight loss a prime example of how surgery can greatly improve someone's functional ability and feeling towards their body. However, body image concerns, including the serious body dysmorphia disorder, can be worsened by plastic surgery and reputable surgeons are always on the lookout for this. While plastic surgery can be life-changing for a number of people, for others, it might risk psychological harm.

Plastic surgery might make you look better but it isn't always good for you. Risks exist, including the risk of dying under anaesthesia. In the battle of the bulge, liposuction might chisel our abs but some studies have shown it has significant effects on our health. Liposuction could alter our metabolism and result in a compensatory increase in fat deposition around our internal organs, which is strongly associated with heart disease and diabetes. This can be reduced with exercise and, of course, research is ongoing, but it does provide food for though. Are we potentially sacrificing our health for the perfect waistline?

Exercise – a cure all?

I prescribe drugs every day. Ranging from medications to unblock clogged arteries to tablets people take for the rest of their life, it's all part of modern medical care. In reality though, I could also write a prescription for exercise. In fact, I do. Getting people moving before and after heart surgery is one of the most important parts of their recovery and future health. The positive effects of exercise are perhaps as important as taking an aspirin every day. Even though we rely strongly on tablets, exercise probably has as many health benefits, as demonstrated in a meta-analysis published in the *British Medical Journal*. However, not everyone takes their tablets and fewer people probably take their exercise prescriptions. While exercise is good for you, it still does not replace medicines; but there is no doubt that, whether you need tablets or not, most of us should be moving more than we currently do.

Tablets are a marvel of modern medicine but exercise is truly astonishing. When you exercise, a number of things happen in your body and these processes are remarkable. Transformations on the outside are really nothing compared to what happens on the inside. Exercise calls on so many different parts of your body, such as your muscles, your cells and your heart, and even short periods of exercise lead to measurable improvements in how all of these organs work. When you exercise, your body's requirements for energy to be delivered to hard-working muscles are up to 50 times higher than when you're resting. When we start exercising, blood is diverted away from our gut and kidneys to the muscles. Our blood pressure goes up a little to deliver oxygen-rich blood, and our lungs work overtime to maintain our oxygen levels so we can power through the workout.

And, after some time sweating, huffing and puffing, our bodies make adaptations that make us fitter and stronger. This means that after even a short period of training, we can outperform our former self and do things we might not have been able to do beforehand. Our skeletal muscles, which drive our limbs to exercise or play sport, grow in size, strength or efficiency and develop more blood vessels to allow better delivery of nutrient-rich blood. Our bodies become expert at using energy, making more energy powerhouses, called mitochondria, inside our cells to power hungry muscles. They become better at using fat as an energy source, leaving untouched our other important energy stores such as glycogen from muscles and the liver. Our hearts can grow a little, get more efficient and pump harder for longer. As you can see, none of the incredible feats performed by our bodies have anything to do with what we look like, they are simply an impressive symphony of our body mechanics.

Exercise is so vital to health that being active, even for short periods a day, drops your risk of dying by 30 per cent. It decreases your risk of heart disease by as much as 45 per cent, making it one of the best treatments for heart disease we have. For instance, if your risk of heart disease was 10 per cent, exercise could drop that to 5.5 per cent. The benefits don't just stop at your heart: research shows exercise reduces rates of breast, lung, colon and kidney cancer. These are the results of maintaining a healthy body weight and also reducing some hormones such as oestrogen and insulin, which might be cancer promoting in some people. Exercise wards off dementia and depression and leads to improved body image and body satisfaction. This is not about weight either. Cardiorespiratory fitness prolongs our lives so much that there is no upper limit: you can't be too fit, according to research. Even if marathon runners, who have more calcium in their heart arteries, have a heart attack they survive it more often than someone without that insane level of fitness.

Despite these benefits, not enough of us are moving and, even if we are, it's not enough. Current WHO guidelines state that we should be exercising at moderate intensity for 150 minutes a week, which is where the commonly heard '30 minutes a day' advice comes from. If you exercise more strenuously, you might need to do just 75 minutes per week. Some experts consider that these figures are merely the minimum of what we should be doing: the more active we are, the more that translates into big health gains. However, with benefits for our health being shown with only 90 minutes of moderate-intensity exercise per week, my own adage is that some is better than none and more is better than some. Even a slow jog for five minutes a day translates into having a healthier heart and dying later. Despite this, globally around 31 per cent of adults aren't getting enough exercise to be healthy; this inactivity is a big target for disease prevention.

There are a lot of reasons why we don't exercise, ranging from that feeling when the alarm goes off in the morning and we simply cannot be bothered, to complex social issues. For women, there is a burden of stereotype about playing sport and being active that can really limit participation. There is a strong concern about how they will be perceived when they're exercising that dissuades them from getting out there. Targeting women through programs or products that appear to champion female empowerment has an uncanny ability to counter the feelings of inadequacy that prevent them being active. There are a multitude of other factors at play here too, including cost, time and access to physically and emotionally safe places to exercise.

In recent years, social media stars and bloggers who endorse forms of restrictive eating have started to downplay the effect of exercise on our health or ability to have a 'bikini body'. This message stems from the finding that 'you can't outrun a bad diet', with catchy sayings like 'abs are made in the kitchen'. Popular bloggers have perpetuated the idea that exercise is not as important as a strict diet. This notion takes known science – the importance of diet – and misreads it to state that exercise is not important. It prioritises how you look over the benefits that come from making sure you participate in a multitude of healthy behaviours.

The downplaying of exercise is not helpful, given that many studies have shown its overall benefits. Exercise and diet are not in direct competition: they are complementary. Exercise has been shown to help maintain weight loss in multiple studies; even if your BMI puts you in the overweight or obese category, being active is still a huge win for your health.

The other important aspect of exercise is that it actually helps us stick to good nutrition and safe eating patterns. Studies have demonstrated that exercise helps us make healthier choices when it comes to food, and that abrupt dieting and calorie restriction in the absence of exercise is tremendously hard to maintain. Modern diets such as cleanses and ketogenic regimens often sell themselves as a magic pill, a five-day cleanse or a keto kick-start. Popular Australian online trainer Ashy Bines has been pushing a keto-kickstart, advertising that you will lose five to eight kilograms in five days. These unsafe dietary quick fixes seem much more attractive than slogging it out on a running track or at a gym and could contribute to the popular notion that diet is king at the expense of a well-rounded, holistic approach to health.

Either way, not many people know too much about the benefits of exercise other than it helps us lose weight. This focus on appearance, on size or on a goal item of clothing can be a hindrance in maintaining not just a five-day cleanse but also our need to have a sustainable and enjoyable lifestyle that includes all the ebbs and flows in our motivation and busy lives. By peddling exercise as a way to get a bikini body, we're again focusing on what is not important; this can be demotivating, lead to dangerous exercise patterns or just set us up to feel we've failed, yet again. But then, since people are more and more inactive, does it really matter what makes us move as long as we get it done?

Breaking down the science of picture-perfect trainers

If you scroll through Instagram, Facebook or a tabloid news site, it's pretty common to see a workout that promises you results you have never ever seen before. A workout that is guaranteed to burn fat, build lean muscle and leave you in the best shape of your life. Each workout has some sort of selling point, aside from the fact that it's the best thing you will ever come across: it's easy to do, takes only a few minutes a day and requires no equipment. Or it's done by a famous model so, therefore, it *must* work. A trainer at a gym I used to frequent is often featured in the news touting the latest and greatest workouts of the year – as if we have learned so much more about the science of exercise in the past 12 months it has completely superseded what we used to do last year. When there is so much miraculous information flying around, you have to stop and ask yourself, what is right and who is just trying to sell me an app?

There is a constant stream of claims made that one exercise is better than another: high-intensity interval training (HIIT) is great but CrossFit is better and so on. Just like the clothes we put on our bodies, fitness and exercise have trends that evolve with the seasons. HIIT is a popular online workout, like the one Joe Wicks sells. So are the circuit classes of Kayla Itsines, the team sport feel of F45 and CrossFit, and the spirituality of yoga. Just like diet tribes, each army of exercisers feels that their workout is the best for health, fitness, physique and generally feeling good about yourself. Proponents back up their claims with before-and-after shots and testimonials or, even better, a short blurb about how this workout has been scientifically studied (or, my personal favourite, 'clinically proven') and is the greatest of all time. That evidence doesn't necessarily exist.

Each of these workouts does have advantages. HIIT, for example, improves fitness and does not take up much time. Running, even for as little as five minutes a day, can reduce your risk of dying by up to 50 per cent, compared with those who never run. Yoga shows beneficial effects on blood pressure, cholesterol, body weight and mood, while resistance or weight training improves bone density and muscle mass. Aerobic exercise, such as running, may be superior to weight training for motivation and body image, while sport, as opposed to exercise, might have similar effects because of the social environment and ability to master a skill. They all have different health considerations: weightlifting doesn't affect your cholesterol levels, running doesn't improve strength or muscle mass, and yoga has little or no benefits for your blood sugar. For any workout to sell itself as vastly superior to anything else that's out there is misleading.

In an effort to make exercise more accessible, popular workouts are marketed as taking only a short time, sometimes as little as a few minutes a day. Joe Wicks is a proponent of just 15 minutes a day. He uses impressive before-and-after photos as testimonials to

What is HIIT?

High-intensity interval training (HIIT) is a type of training that
intersperses periods of intense anaerobic exercise with
lower intensity recovery periods. Its popularity seems to
stem from the ability to cram a workout into a short space of
time; it also has physical benefits for cholesterol, blood
pressure and insulin sensitivity. The downside is that,
because you are flogging yourself hard, you might start to
struggle with motivation. Research has also tended to focus
on short-term outcomes and, unfortunately, men seem to
derive more benefit from HIIT than women. All in all though,
it shows some promise, which is why it feels as if every
trainer on the planet considers it the best thing since sliced
bread. (Although I don't imagine many of them actually eat
sliced bread on account of all the carbs.)

the effectiveness of his *Lean In 15* workouts. Research into these
ultra-short workouts and HIIT routines shows health benefits such
as a little bit of weight loss and some fitness. My philosophy of
exercise has always been to just *do something*; the science seems to
say that even short workouts, if done safely, can improve your
health. What these workouts claim to do for your physique though,
is a big stretch. Some studies have shown that HIIT workouts only
lead to around 1.3 kg of weight loss. However, if you like HIIT and
the short workouts make exercise more accessible, then please go
for it.

In 2018 the US Department of Health and Human Services
released the second edition of *Physical Activity Guidelines for*

Americans. The very first line of their recommendation was that adults move more and sit less, and that some physical activity was better than none. The guidelines then went on to explain that adults should aim for 150 minutes a week of moderate-intensity physical activity, less time if they did more intense activity. They also promoted strength activities for muscle and bone health. However, their major take-home point was: if that's more than you can do right now, then just do what you can. Even five minutes of physical activity has real health benefits. Unlike the hordes of Instagram trainers or gyms telling us that one workout is superior to another, these scientifically grounded guidelines make no such claims. We just need to get moving and how we do it doesn't matter. Inactivity is a bigger problem than not doing the latest abdominal exercise. Exercising needs to be achievable, not another benchmark that is just too easy to fail.

Providing some kind of workout that people can follow is not a bad thing; however, making claims that one workout is better than another could be misleading. If a trainer is selling you your best-looking body/abs/butt ever, that is just garbage. On top of this, they shouldn't be advising you on nutrition, lifestyle or psychology, as it falls well outside their expertise. Everyone's body is different biologically and will respond to each workout differently. We already know that getting people to move to look good is not a useful motivator; we need to aim for health before looking like a before-and-after on Instagram. What *is* definitely important though is moving, in any way, for as long as you can, and to make that something that you can keep up, do safely, master and enjoy. Anything else is just icing on the cake.

How bikini bodies make us move

Whether it is Itsines, Wicks, or the woman down the street, there is no denying the lure of the transformation post. Itsines, for example, has been very vocal in her desire to get women moving for their health and uses women in bikinis to act as the impetus for change. Of course, photos of smiling women in bikinis probably sell a lot of subscriptions to her exercise programs. The number of people worldwide who do not do enough exercise is cause for concern and women in particular are prone to not being active enough. You could therefore argue that as long as people are moving, does it matter why? What's the harm in being motivated by swimsuits?

When researchers surveyed over 2000 American households, 94 per cent of them knew that exercise was important for health, but we don't see that knowledge being translated into action. What we're missing is the link between knowing we should be more active and actually doing it. Motivation to exercise is being studied, but our current approach seems to be similar to my gym trainer's: force them. For years, we have been simply telling people to exercise because 'it's good for you' or to achieve some arbitrary target such as 10,000 steps a day.

There are two broad theories as to why people lack motivation to exercise. The first is a lack of interest in prioritising exercise over other activities. In a large European research study, 40 per cent of subjects said that exercise didn't interest them and they would rather do other things with their spare time. In a world when we're all busy, carving out 30 minutes a day to exercise isn't always straightforward and can mean sacrificing other things, such as family time. In addition, some people shy away from exercise because they don't feel fit enough or good enough at that activity or sport.

Some of us can grind out our exercise despite the fact that we really don't feel like it or don't have time. A number of people exercise because they feel they *have* to, rather than want to. As we discussed earlier, this external motivation may well vanish with time, resulting in a lack of follow-through or commitment. Appearance is a very strong external motivator and is often openly or sub-consciously communicated by social media fitness influencers or used with other workout programs. A number of psychological studies have looked at the effect of this and the research tells us that exercising or dieting for the sake of our appearance leads to more body dissatisfaction, disordered eating and lower self-esteem. One Australian study found that appearance-based motivation to exercise is also associated with a strong desire to avoid gaining weight, which may lead to guilt. Guilt or shame are factors we might think motivate exercise, but it now seems that wanting to look good can lead to *less* exercise, not more.

When researchers showed a group of Australian women 'fitspiration' (fitness + inspiration) images of athletic-yet-thin bodies, although the women thought they looked inspirational, it led to increased body dissatisfaction and did not prompt any actual exercise. In fact, the link between body dissatisfaction and exercise may be so problematic that research has shown exercise makes people with significant body dissatisfaction feel *worse* about their bodies rather than better. This is astounding, because we generally think of exercise as good for body image. Essentially, being motivated to exercise by appearance does not seem to lead to safe, sustained habits and is problematic for mental and physical health.

One of the common ways we see modern exercise programs motivate us is by the use of comparison posts. As we've noted, Itsines' Instagram documents the progress, often called a 'journey' or a 'weight-loss journey', by using before-and-after pictures. The after photo is aspirational and often shows a really exceptional physique earned through a huge commitment. Expert researchers in this area were divided on the effectiveness of such a motivator; some say it can be aspirational because these transformations can happen in normal people rather than celebrities, so the goal is more achievable. Others are cautious to call them good motivators because of the emphasis on appearance and weight loss, which may work initially but are still extrinsic motivators.

Some people who put up aspirational posts may genuinely wish to motivate, while others do it for fame, likes or money. People are sceptical of motivational posts by corporations or businesses and are more likely to feel motivated by an individual, especially if they see a similarity. Other studies have shown that while some people are motivated to exercise by seeing someone who looks better than them, or someone they think is doing better than them, others find this unhelpful, even harmful. Universally though, the more exercise-related social media posts you're exposed to, the more concerned you are likely to be about your weight.

We need to educate posters and viewers to use this motivation safely and with caution. It's important as social media users or consumers of any kind of fitness trend that we look critically at what we're being sold. A picture is quite literally a snapshot of someone's life and habits and tells us nothing more than what they looked like at that particular time. It bears little relationship to their actual fitness, the program they follow, their genetics, its applicability to us or even the picture before it was photoshopped. Most importantly, it does not at all correlate with their health.

Harnessing motivation

For years, we've tried to force, shame or bribe people into exercising – with overwhelmingly bad results. Motivation is a vital tool, but the trick is to tap into our internal motivators. When we have intrinsic motivation, we do an activity because we find it inherently satisfying. We enjoy ourself and feel a sense of accomplishment, leading to long-term commitment rather than just hanging in there for an extreme eight-week program. Exercising for our health is a powerful internal motivator if we can tap into it, because health and wellness are of immense value to everyone.

Dr James Dimmock PhD, an exercise and sports psychology researcher at the University of Western Australia, researches how to access our own internal motivation to exercise – he says this is important in order to stimulate healthy behaviours. Again, intrinsic goals such as being social, achieving personal growth and improving our health are vital at keeping us moving, whereas seeking power, wealth or beauty are not essential to our development or wellbeing and, in fact, get in the way of these things. It's important to strip back our goals and get to a place where the motivation is intrinsic, Dr Dimmock says, adding that it's important that we are honest with ourselves about this. It's no good saying you're motivated by health but what you really want is a better butt to look good in jeans. However, he says it is possible to buy into your own self-talk and that perhaps telling yourself that exercise is good for health or other intrinsic reasons can be cultivated with time. In this sense, while it would be great if we were all able to put aside superficial, extrinsic motivators, if we're able to start there but develop something more meaningful, we may be able to tap into the power of self-determination, fulfilling our psychological needs and accessing intrinsic motivation.

These psychological theories are interesting; even without a background in psychology you can probably appreciate that focusing on your appearance can be counterproductive. In a world that is preoccupied with beauty, battling against the message that you need to exercise to look better is challenging. Transformation Tuesday, Instagram influencers and eight-week challenges are not going anywhere.

Drop and give me 20

Like my gym trainer who tortured us with burpees, motivation can come from those who give us exercise advice and instruction. A number of people work out with a trainer or in a group environment for the stimulus and accountability. Just like the motivation that we give ourselves, what is given to us by personal trainers really affects how much we exercise.

The means by which the message to exercise, or to keep going when we're sweating hard, is conveyed to us is important. The way people in authoritative positions communicate with us can affect our psychological fulfillment. Communication styles that acknowledge our autonomy and barriers, offer meaningful choices and show a genuine interest in our welfare are more likely to engage the self-determination that is important in sustaining a behaviour. On the other hand, when the communication is prescriptive, lacks choice, denounces our feelings or hinges on guilt, it doesn't support our psychological needs and may not lead to exercise. Researchers in this area are looking at ways to apply this motivation everywhere from the doctor's office to the physiotherapist to the gym in an effort to better engage people in lifestyle change.

It's actually quite common for instructors in group exercise classes to adopt a style of communication that is more tough than supportive. This seems to stem from a belief that applying pressure and maintaining control over people will make them work harder. Research has shown that this isn't the case and, over time, a number of people drop out of such classes. However, when exercise instructors are shown how to use a style of communication that is more conducive to empowering people's own psychological needs, exercisers feel more autonomy and are more likely to keep coming back. In addition, the instructors themselves feel they're doing a better job.

Another issue is a focus on appearance. Talking about how great a body part will appear, or how good we will look in time for summer, does not tap into our basic psychological needs at all. Motivational tactics that include making comments on appearance are associated with poor mood and worse body satisfaction. Conversely, when instructors focus on function by remarking on how strong we're getting, it leads to the reverse. These seem to lead to better health behaviours in both diet and exercise.

That's not to say that the bootcamp yelling routine doesn't work for some people. It used to work for me when I was younger because I saw it as an opportunity to prove the trainer wrong. Now, I have better things to do with my time than be yelled at by people in lycra.

Appearance-based motivators for exercise and weight loss take the focus away from what's really important, and that is our health. Our obsession with looking good might sustain exercise for a short period of time but it is also associated with bad psychological outcomes such as poor body image. It's noble to imagine fighting the multi-billion-dollar fitness industry and the people who benefit from it, such as the ever-growing number of personal trainers. But this isn't going to change any time soon, not without some sort of regulation from government, which is commercially unviable so not likely to happen. But we *can* question everything we see online and expose ourselves to healthier motivation style, one that has nothing to do with bikini bodies. That is a challenge I know we can *all* rise to.

Chapter 5

EATING DISORDERS: THE UNBEARABLE LIGHTNESS

'Nothing tastes as good as skinny feels.'

KATE MOSS, 2009
(SHE RETRACTED THIS STATEMENT IN 2018)

Content warning: please note that this chapter contains discussions of eating disorders, which some people might find distressing or triggering. If you need advice or would like to talk to someone after reading this, a list of resources is available at the end of the chapter.

Full disclosure: I am not an eating disorders expert. My memories of exposure to eating disorders in the course of my medical career span back to my days as a medical student on the teen ward at the paediatric hospital. The girls who had been hospitalised were painfully thin, wearing baggy tracksuit pants in the warm Australian weather, with nasogastric tubes funnelling nutrition directly to their stomachs. The doctors and nurses all spoke of them with a sense of nihilism, understanding the challenges of treating their disease. They tried and tried but these girls could not be reached; they were trapped by their disease. In desperation, I was once tasked with talking to a girl with anorexia in the hope that I could 'reach her' as though, being a young woman myself, I might have some mystical power to understand her turmoil and magically inspire her to start eating. I'm sure the team didn't really think I held the key, but the frustration of the medical workers that they could not save these girls was palpable.

In the course of delving into the broad range of issues about our messed-up relationship with healthy behaviours, I approached a number of experts, including researchers, doctors, dietitians and psychologists. In looking at dieting, exercise and the effects of the media and society on our health, it's impossible to ignore eating disorders as a possible serious outcome of this madness. So I reached out to a different kind of expert in the field of eating disorders and that was one of my very dear friends.

It's common knowledge among our friendship group that she had a serious eating disorder. We'd had glimpses of the tumultuous years she and her family had experienced, and kept a subconscious group eye on her at times we considered could make her sick again: her wedding, pregnancy, before surgery, or the time she worked as a psychiatric registrar and relived the limitations of the mental health system's ability to treat young people in need. I sat down with her at five months pregnant and listened to her story as she told it in its entirety for the first time. Sitting on the couch opposite my brave friend, I tried not to cry or be angry with the way our society fails vulnerable people who can be so determined not to eat that it costs some of them their life.

You know those kids who look a few years older than they are?

Taller and bigger? That was my friend Tara. From a young age, although there was absolutely nothing wrong with her, even strangers would comment on her body. Not in a bad way, but it seemed that her body, even as a child of nine years old, was for public consumption. It wasn't until an injury put a stop to her sports pursuits at age 12 that someone decided to mention weight loss. A well-meaning physiotherapist pointed out to Tara's mother that, since she wasn't exercising as much, her weight was sneaking up and she ought to put a stop to it. Tara developed a 'secret power' – making herself sick – and remembers doing that after eating her cake on her thirteenth birthday. While others remember parties and presents, Tara remembers the vomiting that gave her control. She was full of cake, and then she wasn't. Suddenly, she had a tool to control her fullness, her weight, bullying at school and any other challenges she faced.

What happened from there pains me. What started as something she hid at home, became something she hid from everyone, and it grew and grew. It degenerated from skipping meals to not eating at all. It became life threatening when she was admitted to hospital, hypothermic because her body didn't have enough calories to maintain her core temperature. It barely had enough nutrition to keep her heart beating. For the better part of a decade, Tara was in and out of hospitals and day programs as her parents battled to keep her alive. Because that's what this was about, keeping her alive. Most hospital admissions only made things worse as she was isolated from her beloved dancing, friends who didn't have eating disorders and school. She learnt from other girls about calories and how to sneakily siphon away the feed from her nasogastric tube in the middle of the night so she wouldn't gain any weight. She endured the cruel nurse who used to refer to the girls with anorexia as the 'EDs' (eating disorders), taunt them with graphic descriptions of pizza and burgers and ask them to guess the fat content of his meals.

For almost ten years, Tara starved herself. As her friend, my heart aches for the pain she must have been going through, which makes this story the hardest thing I have had to write. That pain quickly turned to anger though when she told me of the times people would congratulate her on her weight loss when she had just started to purge. I was infuriated at how many people felt they had the right to comment on her body; in fact, on all of our bodies, as if it were just a normal part of human interaction without realising how dangerous it can be. I am despairing that nowadays you can learn online how to have an eating disorder, thankfully something not available to my friend back then. Even if you don't have a full-blown eating disorder, you can now flick through social media and find tips and tricks to help you fit into your jeans, a bikini or a wedding dress from people who *do* have eating disorders. I mean, what better way to lose weight than learn from someone who is making a career of starving themself? At least you know it works. Depending on where you live and how much money you have, treating an eating disorder can be expensive, unsuccessful and, sometimes, even make things worse. I wonder how many of the girls I saw on the teen ward were cured of their illness. I wonder how many survived.

For a long time, the media, social media and diet culture have been heavily criticised for causing eating disorders. A few decades ago, blame was levelled at waif-like models such as Kate Moss and other girls who walked the runway on legs so thin that the crowds gasped. Now, as my friend Tara says, the internet and social media have taken over from fashion magazines as the how-to manual for starvation or purging. A lot of the advice around our health makes us feel bad, spend too much money, and damages our mental and physical health. For others that damage can be far worse. How much does our obsession with thinness drive eating disorders?

What are eating disorders?

Eating disorder is a term that gets thrown around a bit but it is not a diet or being fussy about what you eat. Eating disorders are psychiatric illnesses with a very strong physical component; they are described in *The American Psychiatric Association's Diagnostic and Statistical Manual of Mental Disorders, Fifth Edition* (DSM-V). Broadly speaking, eating disorders are characterised by a 'persistent disturbance of eating that impairs health or psychosocial functioning', which is a technical way of saying that your eating is so disturbed it makes you sick, physically, mentally and socially. The DSM provides a set of criteria that have to be met in order to get that diagnosis. The criteria are revised and debated with each new iteration of the psychiatry bible. According to DSM-V, there are several recognised categories of eating disorders, including anorexia nervosa, bulimia nervosa, binge-eating disorder and unspecified eating or feeding disorder. These are the ones that have a link with dieting, weight loss and eating problems in women, girls and adolescents.

The history of anorexia-like eating begins with descriptions of religious fasting in the pre-Christian era. Women would starve themselves in the name of religious piety; it was sometimes referred to as *anorexia mirabilis*. English physician Richard Morton first published descriptions of patients with anorexia in 1689; this was followed by the publication of more such case descriptions over the following 200 years. In 1873 Sir William Gull, one of Queen Victoria's personal physicians, published a paper which coined the term *anorexia nervosa*, describing a number of cases along with their treatment. More than a century later, in 1978, German–American psychoanalyst Hilde Bruch published *The Golden Cage: the Enigma of Anorexia Nervosa*, which identified highly intelligent middle-class girls as the most common sufferers of the disease.

Although they have been around for centuries, eating disorders became much more visible during the twentieth century. Bulimia was described among some of the wealthy in the Middle Ages, who would vomit during meals so they could consume more food. The first clinical paper on the disease was published in 1979.

The death of singer Karen Carpenter, a huge star of the 1970s and 1980s as one half of The Carpenters, brought anorexia out of doctors' surgeries and into the open. She died of heart failure caused by complications relating to anorexia; her death prompted widespread media coverage of the disease and its deadly toll.

Anorexia is probably the most well-known disorder and affects around 1 per cent of women and less than 0.5 per cent of men. These figures could be low because anorexia is under-diagnosed. Sufferers can be missed, they may conceal their behaviour, or we simply call them skinny. More recent research has also shown that people do not have to be severely underweight to have an eating disorder, sometimes allowing them to go unnoticed for long periods. Anorexia tends to start in mid-adolescence but it can begin at any time, which makes it tricky to spot. Interestingly, anorexia in boys is more common in childhood for reasons nobody really understands. For most people with the disease, anorexia's hallmark is extreme weight loss and its severity is calculated using BMI. Although BMI is often misleading, in this instance it can be useful to determine how unwell someone is. People with anorexia can sometimes starve themselves through extreme restriction of their food, or even binge and purge or exercise excessively and compulsively. In addition to the extreme weight loss, people with anorexia have an intense fear or aversion to weight gain and a seriously misplaced idea of how their body looks. We might see jutting bones, while they focus on areas they perceive as fat.

Bulimia nervosa is slightly more common than anorexia, occurring in around 2 per cent of women and 0.5 per cent of men, although it too might be under-diagnosed. Bulimia manifests as episodes of binge eating, when the sufferer eats massive amounts of food in a short space of time. They feel they have no control over this eating and then, in order not to gain weight, they resort to compensatory behaviours such as vomiting, taking laxatives or diuretics (medications that make you pee), or periods of fasting. The mention of fasting particularly rang alarm bells for me. How many people do you know have been on a fast after over-indulging? Like anorexia, bulimia is graded by severity, with specialists looking at how many times the sufferer 'purges' or compensates in a week, ranging from 1–3 for mild to over 14 for more severe. Sufferers are highly influenced by their weight and shape.

Binge-eating disorder is a new addition to the current version of the DSM-V and tends to occur in midlife. With binge-eating disorder, people eat more food than normal more quickly to a point when they feel uncomfortably full. They experience a loss of control and intense feelings of distress. I know many of us can easily think of a time we stuffed ourselves, but this isn't the same as just eating too much Christmas dinner. Neither is it having a 'cheat meal', a popular diet strategy that promises to reset your weight-loss goals and provide some relief from constant chicken and broccoli. Studies have demonstrated the mass calorie consumption that comes with a cheat meal differs strongly from bingeing because it doesn't bring that same psychological distress. The anguish and loss of control while bingeing is what sets this disorder apart. It also has to happen at least once a week for at least three months. The difference between binge-eating disorder and bulimia is that sufferers don't compensate for their massive food intake. This means that binge-eating disorder has a much higher rate of obesity and associated illnesses, such as diabetes.

The other diagnosis is a bit of a mixed bag: unspecified eating or feeding disorder. This is applicable to people who have significant distress, symptoms (physical and mental) but don't quite meet the criteria for the more specific disorders. This is estimated to affect 3 per cent of people and describes disorders such as atypical anorexia nervosa with which the sufferer has a normal BMI.

There are other eating disorders, such as avoidant–restrictive food-intake disorder, with which there are serious food-restriction issues but, unlike the other illnesses, there is an absence of body image concerns. At their core, eating disorders like anorexia and bulimia are centered around food, eating and body image. They lead to ritualised and highly driven behaviours of dieting, purging, compulsive exercise and binge eating. After a while, people with eating disorders spend more and more time on these disruptive behaviours and become more and more preoccupied with food.

As the illness continues to take hold, their lives – and usually the lives of those around them – become increasingly impaired; their regular life drops away, consumed and replaced by their illness. Research into those who have eating disorders has shown serious impairments in their quality of life and a negative effect on their families.

Eating disorders are thought to be becoming more common for reasons nobody quite understands. It could be that we're looking for them more or that more people are truly unwell. What I find particularly disturbing is that one of the limitations to understanding how common they are is that so many elements of eating disorders are normal in our society. Skipping meals, diet pills, extreme calorie restriction, purging and body image obsession are all ways we describe what we're doing to lose weight to be 'summer body ready'. Dangerous dieting is so pervasive, so normal and so accepted that we don't understand these behaviours should be considered a barrier to our health and wellbeing.

Recovery rates for these various illnesses tend to show that those with anorexia experience a full recovery 40 per cent of the time and a partial recovery another 40 per cent of the time. For those with bulimia, recovery rates are thought to be over 50 per cent. For binge-eating disorder, these rates can be even better. Before we start patting ourselves on the back, though, it is estimated that as few as 22 per cent of Australians with eating disorders are actually getting medical help. Twenty per cent of people with an eating disorder will die from their illness. And particularly sobering is the fact that suicide is the leading cause of death in those with eating disorders. They are 31 times more likely to commit suicide; it's the most lethal mental illness.

Along the way, the people with this severe psychiatric illness also suffer a litany of serious medical problems. These read like a medical textbook and can include problems with skin, nails and hair, bleeding on the eyes (subconjunctival haemorrhage) from vomiting, dental issues, dry mouth, bad breath and dangerous changes in the composition of the blood, including low potassium which places the heart at risk. People who purge by vomiting develop a 'chipmunk' face due to growth in the glands of their cheeks to make saliva: they're working overtime to keep the mouth moist and healthy in the midst of all the vomiting. In those who use laxatives, the damage to the intestinal function can be permanent. Those with anorexia suffer some very serious heart problems including bradycardia, an abnormally slow heartrate, low blood pressure and a kind of shrinking of the left ventricle of the heart. People with binge-eating disorder often suffer from obesity, diabetes and their various complications.

Treating eating disorders has a dual focus on the person's physical health and also the challenging and sometimes immutable psychological processes that spawn them. Treatment can include meal plans, nasogastric feeds that pass liquid food via a tube directly from the nose to the stomach, and inpatient hospital admissions. Psychiatric and psychological care focuses not only on the patient but also on the family. Patients with eating disorders need a big, specialised, experienced team, which is sometimes hard to access. Private clinics around the world charge large fees, while publicly funded healthcare can struggle to keep up with looking after them. Having cash and an education means you are more likely to get treatment, but this leaves a large number of sufferers exposed and overlooked.

It's important to keep in mind that having an eating disorder is so much more than being very skinny or having issues with food, taking a diet too far or not being able to control your eating. Eating disorders are a life-changing and at times life-threatening diagnosis. They were once considered to be the sole domain of ultra-thin, wealthy, white western women, but are now found around the world across every social, economic and educational demographic. Even people in larger bodies can have eating disorders such as anorexia; we need to broaden our minds so that everyone gets the treatment and compassion they deserve.

Diabulimia

Diabulimia is not an official diagnosis; you won't find it mentioned in any manual of psychiatric disorders. It is, however, a term that has been coined as a portmanteau of 'diabetes' and 'bulimia' to reflect the large number of people with type 1 diabetes who manipulate their insulin dosage to stay slim or lose weight. In type 1 diabetes, the pancreas does not produce enough insulin, which leads to dangerously high blood-sugar levels. We treat this by having the patient check their blood sugars and self-administer insulin by injection several times a day. One of the unusual side effects of injected insulin is that it promotes weight gain. But not keeping the blood sugar tightly controlled with insulin leads to some very serious complications such as heart disease, infections, kidney failure, limb loss and vision impairment.

By incorrectly dosing their insulin, usually lower than it should be, patients lose weight. In fact, one of the ways diabetes can present is with weight loss. Research has shown that those with type 1 diabetes are two to three times more likely to have an eating disorder; an astonishing 37 per cent of girls and women with the illness have disordered eating, eating disorders or manipulate their medications, referred to as 'diabetes compensatory behaviour'. What's also concerning is that the risk of death in these diabetics is three times higher than in those without a disorder.

Research has looked at the reasons why people with this serious disease can go on to develop an eating disorder with such profound health effects. From their first diagnosis, diabetic patients learn a lot about food, with lists of what to favour and what to avoid and, of course, 'good' foods and 'bad' foods. This is thought to lead to a preoccupation with food that can play into an eating disorder. Other research has focused on the fact that people with a chronic illness can feel a loss of control and a sense of not belonging; this can be alleviated by controlling the body through an eating disorder. And body image concerns are just as common in diabetics. It's an interesting mix of factors that leads to these people risking their health.

Eating disorder or disordered eating?

Disordered eating is eating in a way that isn't quite enough to warrant a diagnosis of an eating disorder, but features an abnormal pattern. It covers a broad range of behaviours, including compulsive eating, binge eating, use of diet pills, vomiting and secretive food consumption. Also on the list is chronic restrained eating, which we know more commonly as dieting. The normalisation of behaviours that are inherently bad for us can mean we don't place as much emphasis on the dangers of disordered eating as we should. The main difference between this and an eating disorder is in the severity and frequency of these behaviours.

The Eating Attitudes Test (EAT-26) asks us to grade statements such as 'I avoid eating when I'm hungry' or 'I eat diet foods'. It's used to screen people who might have an eating disorder and is one of a handful of tests used in clinical settings and research to look at irregular eating patterns. The score determines whether someone merits further investigation for an eating disorder. There isn't a cut-off that tips us from disordered eating to eating disorder, mainly because they share many common features. In some research studies people who don't quite have an eating disorder score as highly on EAT-26 as those with a formal diagnosis of anorexia.

Does disordered eating lead to eating disorders, like a stop-off on the way to a full-blown problem? In some cases yes, but not always. While disordered eating and dieting disorders seem to be on a spectrum, it's probably not helpful to treat only when there has been a formal diagnosis of a full eating disorder. Doing so belittles the harm that disordered eating can do to our physical and mental health. A diagnosis of an eating disorder by the standard criteria doesn't capture everyone who is exposed to harm by their food, exercise and underlying psychology around food and body image. Disordered eating can absolutely worsen to a point at which the sufferer, with deteriorating physical and mental health, is diagnosed with some form of eating disorder. Given how prevalent disordered eating is – current figures of around 20 per cent are probably an underestimate – even without a label it inflicts a lot of damage.

Why do we get eating disorders?

I remember at 15 years old being told during PE class to line up, take off our shoes and file into the gym where our height and weight were recorded. They weren't looking for people who were too big; it was to screen for eating disorders. A girl in the year below me had just been hospitalised for anorexia so the school decided to be proactive in a way that was probably not that helpful. But we did fit the profile of the typical sufferer: middle-class, white teenage girls. I remember at the time feeling highly self-conscious that our bodies were being judged and measured.

What we know now is that that this 'typical' picture of someone with an eating disorder misses many people. We were being assessed for being 'too skinny' but eating disorders happen to all kinds of bodies from different races and social classes, including males. My school also assumed that, once one girl had been diagnosed, we would fall like dominoes; while your peer group does influence your behaviour, it's a simplistic view of how these disorders develop.

There is never one single simple cause for developing an eating disorder. They arise in people who are vulnerable and are also exposed to other risks. Research suggests that emotional distress sits at the centre of this: the eating disorder becomes a way of coping with that suffering. There are also certain personality traits, such as perfectionism, neuroticism and avoidance, that are seen more commonly in those with anorexia and bulimia. On top of that, the social and cultural experiences we have can then tip the balance. The way we value thinness or muscularity can be triggering for vulnerable people. Women who internalise an ideal and apply it to themselves are more likely to develop an eating disorder. We need to care about the consequences of poor body image because it is strongly associated with eating disorders.

We need to know more about anorexia, bulimia and disordered eating because of how terrible they can be to live with. Research has looked at the causes of these illnesses and how sufferers can recover. Specialised brain MRIs have shown some possible differences in the pathways connected with reward or in the ability to override motivation to eat and even a disconnect with physical symptoms, concrete thinking styles and a difficulty with emotions,

---

What to watch out for – SCOFF

London's St George's Hospital has developed the SCOFF questionnaire, which asks these five questions to determine if someone is at risk of an eating disorder. Score 1 point for every yes answer.

* Do you make yourself sick because you feel uncomfortably full?
* Do you worry you have lost control over how much you eat?
* Have you recently lost more than 6 kg (1 stone) in a three-month period?
* Do you believe yourself to be too fat when others say you are too thin?
* Would you say that food dominates your life?

A score of 2 or above indicates that anorexia or bulimia is likely. This test has been examined by researchers and found to be very reliable for detecting problems.

---

which is called alexithymia. This could explain why sufferers use their behaviours (subconsciously, of course) to avoid dealing with their emotions. The brain of someone with anorexia might even have a muted response to the taste of food. We could even see something called epigenetics at play, when our genes change the way they instruct the body to work after a particular event. This research could provide more clues about how these illnesses happen and how we can treat them.

Dieters are prime targets for developing an eating disorder. The National Eating Disorders Association report states that 35 per cent of so-called 'normal dieters' develop disordered eating; of that group, 20–25 per cent develop an eating disorder. Australian research shows that women and girls who are severe dieters (those who miss meals, purge or use diet pills, for example) are 18 times more likely to develop an eating disorder than their peers. Obviously not everyone who goes on a diet gets sick, but the restriction or purging has to start somewhere. It makes sense that severely limiting what you eat can escalate to limiting food to a point that is life threatening.

Who is to blame?

Although fashion magazines and models have been around for many years, young women now access the vast majority of their fashion content on the internet and via social media. The fashion industry, along with the diet industry and the media, have been heavily criticised for their role in promoting unhealthy body ideals. Many experts have gone so far as to hold them responsible for eating disorders and our often broken relationships with food and our bodies. The development of disordered eating and eating disorders is a complex problem, and the media, wellness and diet industries aren't innocent parties. To what extent, though, does our constant bombardment with tiny bodies actually cause eating disorders?

Psychologically speaking, we are presented with countless images of thin women we're supposed to want to look like. Research has shown that models are taller, weigh less and have smaller waists than the average woman, and WHO reported in 1998 that 66 per cent of professional fashion models were underweight by BMI standards. We're already facing an uphill battle to emulate these women: biology alone means that very few of us will ever have the figure of a Victoria's Secret model. This predestined failure results in body dissatisfaction and self-objectification, when we consider our bodies only to be admired for how attractive or sexual they are. We constantly monitor our attractiveness and not much else. The more often we are exposed to sexualised images or thin ideals, the more likely we are to self-objectify and be dissatisfied. Body dissatisfaction is linked to unhealthy dieting, less physical activity, psychological distress and even disordered eating.

The diet industry has long been criticised for causing eating disorders. Dieting is reasonably well known to cause eating disturbances, which can precede disorders. Reducing the amount of dieting should lead to healthier eating patterns since it is associated with both eating disorders/disordered eating and obesity. But it's been hard to prove conclusively that diets lead to eating disorders. For example, binge eating and bulimia might actually benefit from the restraint that comes from diets. Research published in *Eating Behaviours Journal* has tied the effect of diets to eating disorders, in the context of recent weight loss and the starting BMI. Women with a normal BMI who then lost weight while dieting were more likely to have eating issues related to dieting. Dieting in adolescence seems to be a particularly high-risk time. In Australia in 2019, a medical study aiming to help kids (yes, children) lose weight by submitting them to 800-calorie 'fasting days' came under fire for setting these kids up for problems, including eating disorders. A growing teenager needs at least double this amount.

The contribution of the media to the topic cannot be ignored. However, although we would like to attribute blame to them, the media is best thought of as a risk factor rather than an actual cause. The media probably impacts most strongly on those people who are already at risk of developing an eating disorder. Research has shown that reading fashion magazines or seeing slim women on TV does correlate with developing a disorder. Happily for magazine publishers, if you buy into that slim ideal, research has shown that you're more likely to use those magazines to get tips and information on how to look like that. Even if you can't possibly achieve it, you're buying more of the magazines. The cynic in me says that publishers probably know that once we're hooked we'll keep buying magazines that promise to help us look like a fitness model. A large study from the *International Journal of Eating Disorders* showed that media consumption and peer pressure are the two drivers of women aspiring to be thin. The risk of the media triggering eating disorders is variable, however – if it was as strong as is often thought, given the ubiquity of fashion images in the media, more of us would have serious eating problems.

Social media has changed all of this, and not for the better. Social media is unique in that it merges two risks for developing an eating disorder: media exposure and peer pressure. Social media has the power to flood us with images of the ideal thin body and then reinforce that ideal by sharing or talking about it, always looking for 'likes'. It takes the traditional media one great big step forwards. Those comments like 'I wish I had your legs' or 'check out your abs', as well as fat talk ('I feel so' or 'look so' fat) just make it harder and harder to ignore the fact that people want us skinny and beautiful above all else. The comparison seems to be central to making us feel bad and leading to problem eating, according to research. If the comparison isn't there, the disordered eating is less likely. It's hard not to compare ourselves to the images we see online because trying to work out where we stand in relation to others around us is almost reflexive. Social media gives us access to thousands of filtered images of people to compare ourselves to, all in the palm of our hand.

They say that comparison is the thief of joy. Human beings are thought to have an innate drive to evaluate ourselves and a psychological theory called 'social comparison theory' looks at just this. We can evaluate ourselves by comparing ourselves to someone seemingly better than us (upwards social comparison) or perhaps worse off (downwards social comparison). Comparing our bodies is easy, especially online and it does indeed seem to be taking away our joy.

Whatever the social media platform, the more time you spend on it, the more likely you are to have psychological fallout. According to figures from the social platforms, a staggering eight million photographs are uploaded every hour onto Facebook, with over 55 million photos and videos uploaded to Instagram every day. Social media is particularly popular with young women, who also happen to be highly concerned with body image and are at the highest risk of disordered eating. On social media, just like in fashion magazines, a single episode of seeing a thin woman might have a fleeting effect on our self-esteem and anxiety levels, but a lifetime of chronic exposure to skinny ideals is probably bad for our psychological health. Viewing idealised images of 'perfect' bodies, even for short periods of time, has been shown in large meta-analyses to increase depression, anxiety and anger, all of which contribute to eating disorders.

A study published in the *Journal of the Academy of Nutrition and Dietetics* sought to pinpoint exactly the link between social media and eating concerns. This paper showed, in a study of 1765 men and women of varying racial backgrounds, that there was a strong relationship: the more you used social media, the more problems you had. In other research into eating problems or body image issues, social media networks such as Instagram are often singled out. Instagram and Snapchat are strongly image based and that inevitably sets off comparisons in your head. Interestingly Twitter, a platform that's far less reliant on pictures, is less likely to produce these kinds of negative outcomes than image-heavy apps.

It's not just those of us browsing social media who are at risk. A study published in the *International Journal of Eating Disorders* looked at women who post fitspirational content on Instagram and found that one fifth of them had behaviours that placed them at risk of an eating disorder. A number of these women compulsively exercised and demonstrated features of disordered eating. These behaviours are normalised – and even celebrated – online.

There is no research 'smoking gun' at the moment to blame Instagram or any other social media platform for eating disorders.

But, just like the traditional media, they're not innocent bystanders. Research generally confirms that using these platforms leads to body dissatisfaction and internalisation of a thin ideal, important factors in the development of eating disorders.

So, social media, alongside mainstream media, has a role to play in the development of our completely screwed-up relationships with food and our bodies. Eating disorders are not overwhelmingly common but they are disruptive and dangerous to our health and wellbeing. However, eating concerns, body image concerns and disordered eating *are* very common and the role that media has to play in them is irrefutable. It's naïve to believe they are the whole reason, but they are not helping any of us with our health and wellbeing. They have a responsibility to do a much better job than they're doing at the moment.

Not everyone with body image issues or disordered eating will develop an eating disorder, but they are likely to be contributors. Social media in particular is creating a perfect environment for these problems. In general, the most vulnerable people are the ones most likely to be affected by social media. One study published in *Appetite* journal looked at both male and female students and showed that even students who were at low risk of developing disordered eating increased their risk the more time they spent on social media. People who are already at risk of an eating disorder can be pushed over the edge by posted images; we need to protect everyone and especially those who are the most vulnerable.

It is hard to police social media and the owners of these platforms are making huge amounts of money from the way things are running right now. It's hard to foresee a massive change in the status quo, such as Victoria's Secret using diverse body types or social media sites policing images to remove those that feed into the development of an eating disorder or general eating issues. The good news is that we may be able to fight back. A systematic review of research concluded that improving our media literacy is a way forwards. It found that improving our ability to assess the messages we're being delivered improves body satisfaction and leads to greater scepticism and greater understanding of the influence of the media and awareness of the media's existence for profit. While there wasn't a strong effect on disordered eating, being able to push back against what we're being sold is a great way to start.

The Fast Track trial: is medical science creating eating disorders?

In 2019, a trial called 'Fast Track to Health' got a lot of publicity. It was to be run out of two Australian children's hospitals on adolescents aged 13–17 years old who were obese. They were enrolled to do either alternate-day fasting of just 800 calories a day, or to go on a general, reduced-calorie diet. The trial was to try to stop these kids getting illnesses like diabetes or heart disease down the track. It was evaluated and approved by ethics boards, a strong safeguard for medical research.

When the trial became public knowledge, the backlash was swift, especially from dietitians, doctors and psychologists experienced in treating eating disorders. Statements from many organisations, including the Australian and New Zealand Academy of Eating Disorders, strongly urged the responsible ethics committee to stop the trial. Dieting, as we have already discussed, does not result in sustained weight loss and may have more health risks than benefits. The risk of developing disordered eating or an eating disorder became the prime target for its opponents. Parents whose children were participating were told only that the risk of an eating disorder was 'low and manageable'. They were not told that dieting could be an important risk factor for an eating disorder and for obesity – the very thing this trial was trying to treat.

The trial was a strong example of how much we value weight loss above all else, to the point where medical professionals were willing to subject children to strict diets that could land them with a lifetime of unintended illness. Dieting is strongly endorsed, even by doctors, even when we've been shown it doesn't work. A hospital-approved research trial might have been unwittingly showing kids how to develop eating disorders that would have an impact on their physical and emotional health for years. Running a research trial is seen as the epitome of science; yet, this trial demonstrated how deeply ingrained dangerous dieting is in our society. I wonder what a trial in which kids are just taught to be healthy and happy, without any weight focus, would look like.

Encouraging eating disorders: the rise of pro-anorexia and pro-bulimia

'Thinspiration', a portmanteau of thin and inspiration, was one of the first online communities of its kind. Thinspiration tends to promote extremely thin bodies, glorify stringent food restriction and provide emotional support for people who want to maintain thinness. There is also a tendency to call eating disorders a 'lifestyle choice' rather than an illness. Because of the potentially dangerous nature and underground existence of these movements it's hard to know much about them, but estimates put these sites at between 200 and 500. The thinspiration hashtag had been used many millions of times.

The content of these websites reflects dangerous attitudes and beliefs that characterise eating disorders. There are strong themes of control, success, perfection, isolation, deceit and solidarity. Not everyone who uses them is severely malnourished, and not all the sites are equally harmful. Those that promote thinspiration and place emphasis on control, sacrifice and solidarity have been shown to be particularly dangerous because they encourage isolating yourself from family and friends who might be able to help. The content includes images that promote body dissatisfaction, dieting and low mood.

Social media sites and internet providers were unusually quick to respond to the dangerous content. In 2012, microblogging website Tumblr banned pro-eating disorder content and banned any users that searched for it. Tumblr posted that 'eating disorders are not lifestyle choices, they are mental disorders that, when left untreated, can cause serious health problems, and at their most severe can even be life-threatening,' along with links and phone numbers to support lines.

Yahoo followed suit, classifying pro-eating disorder content as self-harm; the hashtags #thinspiration and #bonespiration were banned by Instagram and Twitter. But people are crafty: it's easy to configure your hashtag to 'th1nspiration', which sneaks under the algorithim radar. In fact, it was pretty easy to search Instagram for 'thinspiration' and find plenty of pro-eating disorder content.

Censorship is vital in my opinion, but it is fraught. Heavy-handed banning of anything risks pushing it underground or strengthening the resolve of the people involved. One paper published in a reputable medical journal even suggested that regulating access to harmful information by authorities such as doctors and website administrators is paternalistic, anti-feminist and unnecessarily controlling, a view I don't necessarily agree with. I acknowledge that forcing these groups underground can be hard, but it's completely wrong to let these harmful websites carry on.

Before the internet, you couldn't really *learn* how to have an eating disorder and it was probably not so easy to access glorification of a serious illness. Now, these websites expose many more people to a culture they can become enmeshed in and basically give a how-to guide to anyone who needs it. They encourage people to avoid treatment and open the floodgates for anyone to pick and choose dieting tips and tricks from people who are unwell.

Even though pro-eating disorder movements are relatively new, diet culture, thin ideals and body pressures are not. These have long existed in our families, our friends, in the magazines we read and in the bodies we see on TV. Social media and the internet just amplify these pressures to look a certain way and give us unprecedented access to damaging content in the palm of our hand. And its reach is far. Social media has taken seriously the issue of pro-eating disorder content; if only it were as pro-active with the vast amounts of equally damaging content on its platforms.

If you need help after reading this chapter, please contact an eating disorder help line in your area: **Butterfly Foundation National Helpline (Australia)**, 1800 334 673, thebutterflyfoundation.org.au. **Beat, Eating Disorders Charity (UK)**, 0808 801 0677, beateatingdisorders.org.uk. **National Eating Disorders Association (USA)**, (800) 931-2237, nationaleatingdisorders.org

Chapter 6

ANTISOCIAL

'Wake up. Inspire. Be Better. Repeat.'

ANONYMOUS

Social media is everywhere. It is becoming unusual to meet anyone who isn't constantly checking their Facebook/Instagram/Twitter feed and actively choosing not to be engaged in the endless vortex of the online world. Originally created to allow people to connect and share stories, social media has grown into a beastly phenomenon. It boasts millions of users around the world and is a mainstay of how we communicate, as well as a marketing tool, research medium and campaign base.

More and more people now access their health information online. Dr Google is a common way for people to research their symptoms, self-diagnose, learn about their conditions and connect with health-care providers or other patients. But it's not just Google or websites where people get information. Social media has become a way of disseminating health information without any need to guarantee your expertise or the veracity of the information. In fact, following some of this online advice could be directly damaging to people's health.

A large group of social media users are looking for health information and they are mainly younger women, including teenagers. In one Australian research paper, more than a third of women aged 15–29 used social media for health information, looking at fitspiration accounts, detox pages and diet or fitness plans. Instagram is popular amongst younger people for fitness and dietary inspiration. Don't think for a second that anyone who makes a profit or accumulates fame from their social media 'wellness' escapades is not aware that this generation is their target audience. This young audience has money and a voice and is ripe for being exploited by the wellness industry.

Research has shown that on Instagram anything purporting to be 'healthy' is usually promoted with beauty and make-up products, inspirational quotes, restrictive diet practices (such as gluten free or low carbohydrate) and sexualised images of both men and women. Because sex sells, even when it comes to your health. A number of these health-related posts are selling products and, in fact, 2 per cent of health posts are selling beauty products. While anyone can post health-related content, a large proportion are personal trainers and models, and also companies who claim to be in the health sector but seem to be selling nothing more than a quick fix for a bikini body.

Health-care professionals such as doctors, nurses, paramedics and dietitians used to shy away from social media because of concerns about how professional they could be online. This has now changed, with increasing numbers having an online presence. Often this is to interact with other health-care workers but a number of doctors share information on social media for the benefit of patients or to spread messages of health and wellness. They also use it to publicise important information about diseases in their field of expertise. It's estimated that in the US around 60 per cent of all doctors use social media professionally. Online campaigns are also created by government or professional bodies and use social media as a vehicle, such as UK initiative *This Girl Can,* or *R U OK* for mental health. Virtually every health organisation or charity has an online presence, as do huge numbers of academic medical journals. Getting health, wellness and medical information out into the world is now viewed as important by everyone. As health-care professionals, I don't think we have a choice about being online: we have to ensure that people get good-quality information, rather than misleading or dangerous news.

Social media is deeply entrenched in modern life but its role in health, fitness and overall wellbeing can be, at best, a double-edged sword, at worst, a full-on disaster. Stories of spurious or outright dangerous use of social media to post health-related information are not hard to find. In recent years, we have seen notorious wellness blogger Belle Gibson and self-styled 'wellness warrior' Jess Ainscough, who both touted the benefits of diet alone in fighting cancer. Gibson was subsequently shown to not have cancer, while Ainscough sadly died of her disease, with media reports saying she sought out conventional treatment just before she passed away. Aside from extreme cases such as this, health-related social media is a pathway littered with misinformation that lacks health benefits and can destroy self-esteem and body image. However, users have acknowledged the motivation, community support and value of some information online. Can social media actually make us healthy or is it yet another thing breaking our spirit and our bodies? Given the large number of people getting dubious-quality health information from social media, it's important we delve into how healthy or unhealthy our social media use can be.

How social media is making us pretty unhealthy

When you scroll through your favourite social media app, there are huge numbers of posts purporting to be all about your physical and mental health. On the surface, they might appear to have your best interests at heart. Everyone from personal trainers to models to health professionals are sharing recipes, workouts and behind-the-scenes looks at how they live their best lives. Sometimes they share with you some personal struggle like their 'weight-loss journey' or a battle with alcohol and too much partying as a way of showing some vulnerability or how they've turned their life around. Even if they're peddling a product, it's sold as being authentic, scientific and, most of all, the answer you have been looking for your whole life.

Beneath the attractive surface of social media is a web of problems. Despite users' best intentions, it's possible that very little of the information on social media actually contributes positively to our health and wellbeing. The biggest concern is that anyone can get on there, say they're an expert and publish information we take note of because they have abs, a huge following, or claim to be an authority. Better yet, they have stumbled upon 'the secret to health and wellbeing' that nobody else has found or is willing to tell you, but luckily they're altruistic enough to share. Anthony William, hand-picked by the pseudoscience mothership that is Gwyneth Paltrow's *Goop*, claims to get his health information from spirits. Yep, ghosts tell him to tell us that celery cures liver disease. (It doesn't.) Just because you've got a million followers, it doesn't necessarily mean you know anything. It is not the same as a nutrition degree or a medical degree or any other expertise. Harvard Medical School isn't handing out an MD to @macrojane99 because she notched up a million followers on Instagram.

One of the most crucial issues with health information on social media is accuracy. Health experts and patients alike are very critical of the sometimes dangerous information that is shared with vulnerable people. What is alarming is that the largest users of health-related social media and its biggest target are young women. Many high-profile so-called 'wellness bloggers' have shared their journeys with illness, including Australian blogger Loni Jane Anthony who 'cured cancerous cells in the cervix' by eating watermelon and charcoal. Journalist and *I Quit Sugar* creator, Sarah Wilson, who has 230,000 followers, claims to have treated her anxiety by completely cutting out sugar from her diet. She followed this up by suggesting that wearing helmets when cycling did not reduce death or injury and used a bunch of quasi-scientific terms in an infamous blog post to assert some degree of scientific or medical knowledge. She garnered a reputation as a health expert because she wrote a cookbook and this somehow resulted in her being an expert in road trauma. Incidentally, compulsory helmet laws in Australia have been demonstrated in real scientific studies to have reduced death and disability from bike accidents – but by all means, let's listen to someone who writes cookbooks instead.

As a doctor, I find this kind of inaccuracy very disturbing. There is no scientific evidence to show that diet alone can cure cervical cancer, and anxiety is such a multi-factorial illness that just cutting out sugar is not a realistic, stand-alone treatment for the disease. There is good science to support the use of bike helmets on our roads and to suggest otherwise could risk lives. People's trust in what these self-styled experts say can lead to misinformed choices as to what is really good for us.

Medical science is far from perfect but our ability to fight disease is better than ever and it is maddening that people would put their trust in an influencer with pretty pictures over a proven cure. In fact, a study published in the prestigious *Journal of the American Medical Association* in 2018 showed that people who use alternative treatments were more likely to forego proven cancer therapy. These people were twice as likely to die from their cancer. We live in a world where anti-intellectualism is at an all-time high and people distrust science but put blind faith in a beautiful person with a smartphone and photo editing software.

It's hard to determine just how much of the information we're being fed is garbage. In some studies that looked at the accuracy of online health information, the amount of good-quality information is thought to be pretty low. In a Facebook group to support people undergoing bariatric or weight-loss surgery, just 22 per cent of the information posted had any scientific or medical accuracy. Nearly a quarter of the posts were too ambiguous or confusing for expert researchers to even work out if they were accurate. Meaning they are so full of it, they're indecipherable.

Blogs, where people can communicate much more content and establish their credentials through a backstory or list of qualifications, could be even more inaccurate. One study looked at posts, not just from personal blogs but from commercial hosts such as Yahoo!, and found that only 16 per cent of the information was accurate – despite that, the vast majority of people who read them rated them 'credible'. Studies have shown that many diet-related blogs are potentially harmful for people with eating disorders; the content is often written by people whose behaviour fulfils the criteria for an eating disorder and the advice is dangerous. In some fitness and diet support groups, analysis has found up to 86 per cent of information to be harmful.

Noticing a rise in 'healthy eating' blogs, Scottish obesity researcher Christina Sabbagh and her team looked at the accuracy of their health information. They analysed nine influencers with large social media followings of over 80,000 and authentication (blue ticks) and combed through the information shared. Just one blogger, a registered nutritionist, passed muster. The remainder failed to provide evidence-based weight management advice, with a number passing their own opinion as fact. Only two of the nine bloggers had health qualifications. Some of the advice included eating meals with as many calories as commercial fast food, yet guaranteeing weight loss. While this study included a very small sample, it does open the door to further scrutiny of what we're being told.

(Pretty) girl power

Even in the realm of social media campaigns backed by reputable sources, things can go awry. The Australian *Girls Make Your Move* campaign was designed to encourage physical activity for girls and women and had all the makings of a worthwhile campaign. It was backed by the government and showcased girls and women of different body types being active. It had the support of science and seemingly good intentions. However, it was subsequently exposed to be just as flawed as other online campaigns when it was revealed to have paid Instagram models to post images tagging the campaign. It drew significant fire since the models were not necessarily promoting healthy lifestyle practices – the point of the campaign. The models had thin/beautiful ideal body shapes that could perpetuate body image issues or unscientific 'health' practices. In order to get the sweet cash for a bikini shot with a message, Instagrammers had to have 10,000 followers minimum. What the campaign organisers didn't bother checking was that some social media influencers paid to share this message were endorsing alcohol or dangerous dieting practices on their accounts.

Not only do we get beautiful photos masquerading as health content, on social media people can promote anything, including substances that are directly harmful. Years of law-making and policy change has allowed many of the world's governments to place restrictions on advertising products that are just plain bad for us, like alcohol and tobacco. On social media though, these can still slip through the cracks despite the fact that cigarettes and over-consumption of alcohol remain leading causes of death and disability. Alcohol companies, like many brands, are increasing their online advertising and young people in particular notice these ads and interact with them by way of following an account or liking posts. Research has demonstrated that, for young people, liking these posts is also often associated with risky alcohol use such as binge drinking.

Mirror, mirror on the wall

Research into social media and body image is still in its infancy and most studies are correlational, meaning it's hard to prove that Instagram causes body dissatisfaction when it could be the case that people who are fixated on their appearance are more likely to use Instagram. 'People are comparing their appearance to people in Instagram images ... and they often judge themselves to be worse off,' says Dr Jasmine Fardouly, a postdoctoral researcher at Macquarie University in Sydney, Australia.

Some research suggested that *who* we compare ourselves to was key. In a survey of 227 female university students, women reported that they tend to compare their own appearance negatively with their peer group and celebrities but not with family members while browsing Facebook. The comparison group that had the strongest link to body image concerns was acquaintances. Dr Fardouly says that people present a one-sided version of their life online. If you know someone well, you'll know their social media feed is highly curated, but if they're an acquaintance you have no other information to go on.

Another study published in 2019 involved showing 195 young women either body-positive content from popular accounts such as @bodyposipanda, photos of thin women in bikinis or fitness gear, or neutral images of nature. Showing the body-positive content to the women appeared to boost their satisfaction with their own bodies.

'Those two things together are starting to build a little bit of a story that there may be some content that actually is useful for body image,' reported Professor Amy Slater, from the University of West England and senior author on this study.

Selfies can be particularly problematic. For a 2018 study, Jennifer Mills, an associate professor at York University, Toronto, asked female undergraduates to take a selfie on an iPad and upload it to either Facebook or Instagram. One group took only one photo and uploaded without editing, while the other group could take as many as they liked and retouch them using an app. The study found that all the subjects felt less attractive and less confident after posting than when they'd first walked into the room – even those who'd been allowed to edit their photos. Some of the participants wanted to know if anyone had liked their photo before deciding how they felt about it.

'There's this rollercoaster of feeling anxious and then getting reassurance from other people that you look good. But that probably doesn't last forever, and then you take another selfie,' said Professor Mills.

Most of the work so far has focused on young women, but research on men is starting to show that they're not immune. A study found that men who reported frequently looking at male fitspo content said they compared their own appearance to others more often and cared more about having muscles. Increasingly, we're discovering that poor body image in men can be damaging to their physical and mental health, which makes these findings especially concerning.

Longer term research is needed, according to Dr Fardouly: 'We don't really know whether over time [social media] has a cumulative effect on people or not.'

Comparing yourself to someone else is bad enough, but when you throw in manipulation or editing of photographs, it adds a whole new level of risk. In 2012, Israel became the first country to legislate that retouched photos must be declared when used in advertising, and fashion powerhouse France followed suit in 2017. The effects of these manipulated photos have been studied; girls often rate the altered images as more attractive than the original. Our phones can automatically beautify us, and we spend so much time altering our appearance that when we look in the mirror, we compare our own reflection to our altered pictures and so dislike our own, authentic reflection. We don't even know what's genuine anymore. How can we meet an ideal that isn't even real? Aside from the fact that it leaves us chasing the impossible, seeing these modified images on Instagram worsens our body image. As we know, negative body image does not bring health.

Why do we buy into these messages when they can be useless or even harmful? One research study into engagement on health-related social media showed that young girls who have an eating disorder or have previously used detox teas or other weight loss or wellness products strongly engage with health posts. What a vulnerable section of the community to be exposed to the inordinate number of unhelpful or harmful messages online. But it seems that in some ways we're all vulnerable to these messages. I like to think I have a scientific mind, a healthy dose of scepticism and a medical degree to protect me from rubbish online and yet I think I am vulnerable too, just like the 15-year-old girl who uses flat tummy teas from time to time. We all are. Social media has a scary hold on a lot of us and the evidence suggests that, whether we use it directly for our health or not, it has a worrying potential to make us sick.

Social media has an uncanny knack of luring us in, even when we question what we're seeing or just know that it's broadly not so good for us. It is so easy to access; all we have to do is reach into our pockets and social media is there, when we're bored, when we're waiting around, or when we should be going to sleep. Then it becomes a habit that is hard to break. This time online then translates to measuring our self-worth, either by comparing ourselves to other people or placing value on the number of likes or comments we receive on our own content. While we're imagining this aspirational life, even though we know it's bad for us or not realistic, we keep on engaging anyway.

Even though we place importance on someone's qualifications or position as an expert, we also buy into how we perceive that person. If we feel that they're relatable, then we are more likely to find them trustworthy. What's interesting is that on social media, we might not place as much emphasis on objective markers of expertise as we do when we meet a doctor, a lawyer or any other professional. Expertise is replaced by our perceived competence of the person selling the message. And we don't necessarily evaluate this competence by the quality of the information or their qualifications. We evaluate their professionalism, their relevance to the message or product they're selling, how many followers they have and even how attractive or positive they are. How many followers someone has doesn't actually tell us anything about their knowledge of the diet they're promoting. But that's how our minds work.

Added to this, social media is one of the biggest marketing tools in our modern society. In fact, advertising budgets that used to be directed to magazines and celebrities are now directed at social media and influencers. While some countries and some social media platforms require users to declare a financial relationship by using the terms 'ad' or 'sponsored', not all posts are declared in this way. It is still sometimes very challenging to work out if a post is an ad, and this can be particularly hard for teenagers who are huge social media users. Kim Kardashian, for example, is often seen to post photos with products that are directed at weight loss, such as teas and smoothies, none of which have any proven benefit for health or weight loss. But the posts are successful, with some research stating that over 80 per cent of people take the opinion of an influencer on board when buying a new product.

So here we have a perfect storm. Social media, which is everywhere, shares inaccurate and at times dangerous information with commercial links to an often vulnerable population. Under the guise of health. And we know this on some level but, like seeing a traffic accident, we can't look away. We still think that social media has something to offer our health and wellbeing. Despite all of its drawbacks, we're seeking out health and fitness motivation online and using the smoothies, teas and abs workouts we see to motivate us into getting healthy. Social media's hold on health and wellness is not going anywhere, and fitspiration is strong proof of that.

Is fitspiration really motivational?

A combination of 'fitness' and 'inspiration', fitspiration is a popular online hashtag that on Instagram alone has tens of millions of posts and grows every single day. Fitspiration, or sometimes 'fitspo', encompasses all kinds of health, lifestyle and fitness posts, representing the current cultural ideal body for both women and men. Women associated with the fitspiration trend are slim but muscular with little body fat, while the men are hypermuscular and very masculine.

Posts that use the fitspiration hashtag include a huge variety of images but there are some frequent themes. Posts often show the women in clothing or workout gear that emphasises their figure or exposes parts of their body, often sexually objectifying. There are even terms for some of these shots, including the 'belfie' – butt selfie. Inspirational quotes are also posted to rev up viewers into taking part in exercise or diets. Statements such as 'The only bad workout is the one you didn't do' encourage people to take personal responsibility for their health. Food shots are also popular, often featuring bright, beautifully arranged ingredients, or meal prep where containers of perfectly prepared, healthy food are displayed for microwaving during the week ahead.

Fitspiration is not dissimilar to the 'thinspiration' term, although it wants to be a move away from the long-held skinny ideal, indicating that this is a healthier approach. This really resonates with some women: it's a way of fighting back against some of the aspirational body types, such as the dominant and widely criticised waif-like model shape of the late 1990s and early 2000s. Sayings like 'Strong is the new skinny' attempt to show that the focus has moved away from restriction and unhealthy practices to a new body type – apparently a much healthier alternative. After all, strong *is* healthy in a lot of people's minds.

This schtick is working. Women seem to derive a huge amount of inspiration from such posts. Research has shown that fitspiration or health-related posts do actually inspire some people to be healthier. They are also praised for sharing new recipes and food ideas, inspiring people to eat healthy diets without having to spend money on a book. Gym memberships could be cancelled and, instead, fitspiration leaders such as Kayla Itsines, Emily Skye and

Tracy Anderson are showing women how to work out at home. These posts strongly advocate personal responsibility and willpower as the determinant in reaching your goals, with statements like 'You just have to work for it or want it badly enough'. And, of course, you're not alone in all this; an important factor for some women is the sense of community that develops from moving in fitspiration circles online. Essentially, fitspiration seems to be simultaneously empowering, fighting unhealthy body shape messages and fighting against ill health. On the surface, all looks good.

Dig a little deeper though and fitspiration has some issues. Accuracy is a problem, as with so many other health-related posts. People who promote a fitspiration lifestyle, workout or diet may post information that is not as healthy as it seems, such as excessive exercise or dangerous diet practices. These fitspiration leaders who have minimal or no qualifications have an online image that gives them credibility in all things health and wellness. Far from staying in their lane, the beautiful bodies behind the fitspiration accounts dish out advice on everything from nutrition to medical conditions. This lack of detailed specialisation draws criticism from health-care professionals such as dietitians and doctors. They are also likely to sell a one-size-fits-all approach to health and fitness – a program that worked for them or some of their clients or followers. This is not how health is attained, because each and every one of us is different, with different needs.

Where the fitspiration movement really starts to get interesting though is when we start to challenge its claims that it's an improvement on what we did before; that not only is strong the new skinny, it's better. It may appear that fitspiration bodies are better for us, but they are usually harder to attain than the previous skinny ideal. To get a body like these influencers requires strict dieting and a consistent commitment to weight training on a genetically predetermined base. For a lot of us, this kind of lifestyle is not going to be achievable: it costs money, takes time and requires a rigorous diet that can be isolating, expensive and sometimes lacking in nutrition. In addition, while you can probably improve your biology a bit, you can't fundamentally change how it is supposed to be; you can work out with every influencer program under the sun, drink all of the protein supplements and still not look like the girl you're trying to copy.

When it comes to body image, fitspiration falls just as flat as any other body archetype. Research suggests that fitspiration images might make you harsher on yourself. In 2017 Amy Slater, of the University of West England, published a study in which 160 female undergraduates viewed either fitspo, self-compassion quotes or a mixture of both, all sourced from real accounts on Instagram. Those who viewed only fitspo scored lower on self-compassion, but those who viewed the compassionate quotes ('You're perfect just the way you are') felt more positive about their bodies. For those subjects who viewed both the fitspo and self-compassion quotes, the benefits of the latter seemed to outweigh the negatives of the former.

Other research published in *Body Image* journal has shown that when we view images of fitspiration ideals, we feel just as bad as when we look at thin body ideals. Fitspiration lacks inclusivity by usually featuring slim, white women; this can alienate anyone who doesn't fit that type. Even if the fitspiration ideal is posted with some body positive or uplifting message, it results in just as much body dissatisfaction as a thin ideal – we look at the picture, not the qualifying comment underneath. The fact that these people are still thin and beautiful while trying to sell health means that we end up feeling bad about ourselves – and that does not make us healthier. One study showed, and this seems to be a recurring theme, that looking at fitspiration images not only makes us feel bad, it also leads to subsequent lower rates of exercise. Fitspiration places a huge emphasis on personal responsibility, conveniently ignoring the biological, psychological, social and economic barriers involved. This can perpetuate the stigma that unhealthy people are simply lazy, which research has largely proven to be untrue.

Yoga is another common fitspiration theme that advocates health and wellness while trying to encompass the mental wellbeing that is an important part of the practice. Research has shown that again, 'yoga bod' is no different to skinny ideals, with women being shown what are essentially still slim women. These images, like much of fitspiration, sexualise the exposed bodies they show, which can lead to body dissatisfaction and all the accompanying health problems.

You can argue that a lot of these posts come from a good place, and I have no doubt some do. Whether they are fitspiration leaders wanting to encourage women to be healthier, or everyday users looking for the support and encouragement of the fitspiration community, social media has something to offer some people, especially when it's done well. But of course, the cynic in all of us will understand there are some who are not altruistic. It is no doubt, a double-edged sword. Social media, when used for health, can have tremendous power; that is just the society we live in. However, it is a force for both good and for the not-so-good. In the arena of health, it's too valuable to let the not-so-good forces win.

Whose fault is it? Responsible posting and responsible use

When it comes to our health and wellbeing, it seems social media isn't helping. Since we won't be closing our Instagram accounts any time soon and social media does have a role to play in our lives, the way forward is to work out how to improve it. So what are we going to do about it? Who exactly is responsible for the content that is shared and how it is used? Who is going to take responsibility to make social media a safer and healthier place? It's an interesting question that experts are trying to get to the bottom of.

You can argue that people posting online have a responsibility to share information that is accurate and be open about their motives for doing so. The best example of this is the requirement for anyone using social media to label a post as an #ad or #sponsored when they are being paid to use or give an opinion of a product. These rules have come into effect in a number of countries, including Australia, the UK and more recently the US, to protect the large number of people who buy products based on the suggestions of their idols. All this does though is tell us that it's a paid post. It gives you no indication to how much they were paid, whether they were paid to say only positive things, if the product actually works or whether it is dangerous.

If people selling products related to health and wellness state that they're being paid to rave about a tea, a workout or some other product, that should encourage the person seeing that ad to pause and think about their opinion. However, these ads still look exactly like regular posts and even with one or two hashtags, sometimes in a sea of hashtags they can be hard to pick. The laws surrounding sponsored posts are an important way to protect people, but they can only do so much. In 2019 Professor Stephen Powis, medical director of the UK's National Health Service (NHS), called for a ban on celebrities endorsing products online saying: 'Highly influential celebrities are letting down the very people who look up to them by peddling products which are, at best, ineffectual and, at worst, harmful.'

In my hometown a 25-year-old woman with an undetected genetic abnormality died after taking training supplements that led to organ failure. It was a terrible tragedy that illustrated how the wellness industry can put our lives at risk. Her death sparked a parliamentary enquiry into the booming supplement industry, which largely falls outside current laws and processes. The inquiry recommended that we overhaul the system to include compulsory education for gym-goers about potential problems with supplements, and education for gym trainers about healthy eating. This is the right thing to do, to fight back and ensure that everyone is safe.

When Belle Gibson was exposed for not having cancer and for allegedly misappropriating charity funds, she was prosecuted not for the false and dangerous information she peddled, but for financial fraud. Australian chef Pete Evans wrote a paleo diet book that included a recipe for a bone broth for babies that was so high in vitamin A, it would have been toxic for his intended audience, possibly even causing death. The book was cancelled at the last minute by his publisher, yet an online version of the book is still available. Even in such extreme and obvious cases, it's incredibly hard to enforce any kind of punishment or even stop such information from getting out to an unsuspecting public. And while

Gibson and Evans believe in what they're saying and what they're selling and that they truly wish to help people, that doesn't mean that it's okay to sell information that is wrong and dangerous.

Trying to get people who use social media to post responsibly might be challenging but that doesn't mean we shouldn't try to do it. There isn't much research around about responsible posting but it is getting some attention. Lately, there has been a call for everyone who uses social media to consider what they're posting and how it may affect people who are seeing what they share. Popular clinical nutritionist Laura Thomas PhD, along with The Rooted Project and Athletics not Aesthetics, are among social media-savvy health-care professionals who have made the call for those who post to be mindful and understand the responsibility that comes with having a reach of thousands or more.

It's important that anyone using social media understands that the content they post may be triggering or have another negative effect on someone viewing it. This means knowing that posting the number of calories you eat or the steps you take could be viewed by someone with disordered eating. It also means understanding the power of a sexualised image that is being used to explain or sell health, but in fact is just a picture of yourself looking attractive. These kinds of photos should never be used to sell health because they're not *about* health, no matter what you write underneath them – they're just pretty pictures. Influencers need to own that, and they need to own the fact that they may be fortunate enough to have a body type that is naturally or easily fitspirational – but not everyone is like that. Because they know that a focus on appearance is associated with poor health outcomes, influencers should be encouraged to move away from the story that they're beautiful and healthy and focus on things such as celebrating what their body can do aside from looking good half-naked. A focus on the functional capabilities of our bodies has been shown to improve body dissatisfaction and even encourage physical activity.

When it comes to the content and accuracy of posts, the advice we hear time and time again from experts in health, body image and social media fields is that people need to stay in their lanes. Social media influencers must understand that, while something might have worked for them or sounds like a good idea, it may not actually be as useful for someone else. They need to be made acutely aware of the damage that can be done by posting information outside their scope of practice. One way of calling this out is by real experts taking up social media to spread accurate and mindful messages. They should challenge the false messages peddled by those who have no idea what they're doing. If you ever need to be motivated to ensure this, remember that the biggest users of social media for health information are teenage girls. For me, that's a huge reason to call out bad behaviour.

It is a two-way street and, as consumers of social media, we have a role to play here too. Policing the unhelpful things that find their way on to social media is not easy. The sheer volume of what is posted and seen every day makes this a near-impossible task. Being aware of the shortcomings of social media is an important tool to prevent us falling victim to the unhealthy messages.

This is a challenge, however, as research has shown that most people don't limit their exposure to potentially harmful content, despite being advised to do so. Part of the reason is that fitspiration or other health-related accounts may provide a socially acceptable example of disordered eating or excessive exercise, all in the name of health. Once again, media literacy is important – when we show people how to question what they're looking at or the mechanics of what goes into a perfect picture, we see improvements in their body satisfaction.

It is hard work undoing a lifetime of messages that beautiful is healthy and we should aspire to a certain stereotype. We know a healthy body image is crucial to the prevention of eating disorders and that media literacy helps us understand that what we see in a photograph is not even a small part of that person's story. Legislation on photo retouching is one way to help this – it might not be as helpful as we would like, but it is a start.

It is important that we arm ourselves against the barrage of negative side effects that can come from social media. Our health deserves our protection; since exposure to social media can impact negatively on our mental and physical health, it's vital that we all play a role in staying safe.

Social media done right – This Girl Can and the power of the online community

It's hard to imagine a campaign with the tagline 'Sweating like a pig, feeling like a fox' would be successful, but it was. In 2015 Sports England released their *This Girl Can* campaign. Women were the target because they are more likely than men to be inactive. This pattern starts early on in life when girls are put off playing sport because they are worried about being judged or find it too male dominated. It's even been pointed out that at a school level, making girls wear dresses or skirts can mean they play less at break times and this then persists throughout life. Women are strongly appearance motivated, even when they exercise or play sport; elite female athletes commonly say they are under immense pressure to maintain a particular body type. The judgement women are subjected to by themselves and other people is keeping them from doing something truly valuable for their health.

This Girl Can is the opposing force to judgement and embarrassment. The ads depict women of different ages, races and body types participating in a wide range of sports and movements. And they look like they are loving it. The ads are distinctly different to what we see in the fitspiration movement: women look happy, they're socialising, there is very little objectification or sexualisation and the emphasis is placed on what they're doing, not what they look like. These images are what fitspiration wanted to be but failed to achieve. I still remember the first time I saw these ads: I felt inspired and I sure as hell wanted to join in.

The campaign really hit home. In the first year after the launch, surveys done by Sports England showed that 2.8 million women aged 14–40 years old had decided to be active after seeing the campaign. Even in Australia, the other side of the world, we saw the campaign and it started conversations and spin-offs such as *Join the Movement*. (Unfortunately, as we know, the Australian government campaign, *Girls Make Your Move*, stumbled when it paid influencers.)

Research that looked at the effect of viewing *This Girl Can* made positive findings. People seeing the ad were more motivated to exercise and felt a higher satisfaction with their appearance. Unfortunately, if they saw a picture of a posed model afterwards, that satisfaction and motivation dropped away. The next step was to help women actually engage in activity by providing tips and recommendations for getting involved; just seeing the images alone wasn't enough. Nonetheless, this ad campaign was an important part of the solution to getting people moving. It was a desperately needed counterpoint to the age of the selfie.

After living in the well-heeled suburbs of Sydney for a number of years, even I had begun to buy into the notion that you can't exercise unless you're wearing expensive workout clothes and are already beautiful to begin with. This pervasive attitude is stopping people from doing something good for their health. While we're so focused on our appearance and our flaws, we're not getting out and getting active, which is a vital part of being healthy.

A focus on ability and function as opposed to appearance and beauty has been demonstrated to be a powerful way to motivate us to be healthy and fight body dissatisfaction. Focusing on what our bodies can *do* rather than what they *look like* can be a protective factor against negative body image. It is an important change in the way we advertise health for women.

Social media has great potential to be useful in sharing healthy messages, resources and information on health and illness prevention when it is expanded to include community support. Some mental health and sun protection campaigns have been very successful, and social media is used to support people with diabetes and obesity and this translates into real, measurable health gains. By following experts in their fields, such as doctors and dietitians, people can gain access to digestible, accurate and helpful health information quickly and cheaply. The benefits for our health in this online world are there, and although they're not as sexy as a bikini model, they're sure as hell a lot better for us.

Social media is not the devil when it comes to health, at least not all the time. It is just a vehicle for a message and we determine what that message is and how we receive it. Some messages that we get on social media are not intrinsically harmful. They are made, shared and interpreted in the context of decades of exposure to messages about our health and our bodies, advertising and all of our internalised thoughts and feelings. To get healthy on social media, we need much more than we've already being given; we need more than images of beautiful bodies. Social media can and should be used to look at health in a way that is scientific, accurate, achievable and inclusive. It should be viewing health in a way that inspires us rather than makes us feel bad. And we should all care about the messages we're seeing; we need to empower and protect ourselves in an online world that is fraught with difficulty but may also hold the keys to our health and wellbeing.

Chapter 7

BODY POSITIVITY

'You don't get the ass you want by sitting on it.'

UNKNOWN

You can't ignore Tess Holliday. She's got this amazing mane of red hair and the clearest skin you've ever seen, partially decorated with an impressive collection of artistic tattoos. She is straight-up beautiful and sassy to boot. Holliday is also 'fat' as she describes it and has been in a place you would never expect to see a fat person. On the cover of a glossy magazine.

American model Holliday is one of the heroes of the growing movement of body positivity. Holliday is not only a highly sought-after model (not just in the plus-sized world), she also created the online movement #EffYourBeautyStandards, a virtual finger in the air to the unrelenting beauty ideals to which women are subjected. This is somewhat ironic because Tess is undoubtedly a beautiful woman, although her social media accounts reveal huge numbers of people leaving disparaging comments about her appearance, largely her weight.

Either way, Holliday is one of a number of women who have

decided to change the way we look at people's bodies, with stunning results. These women of different shapes and sizes, ethnicity, gender, sexual orientation and ability are making an effort to shift public perceptions away from the traditional ideal of beauty. With a lived experience of discrimination, eating disorders and strict diets, they are on a mission to help people everywhere love their bodies.

Australian mother, writer and film producer Taryn Brumfitt is at the helm of the infectious *Body Image Movement*. Created after Brumfitt shared a before-and-after picture with a difference, she too wants women to love their bodies. Once a dedicated body builder, she decided to change her attitude to her body and eliminate restrictive dieting and exercise programs when she realised the effect they were having on her pre-adolescent daughter. She shared a Facebook post of her 'before' shot, on stage in a bikini with a physique many people aspire to. The 'after' shot was Brumfitt naked, with the rolls of her tummy visible. The picture went viral and was shared around the world to positive fanfare.

Brumfitt crowdfunded, produced and directed her debut documentary, *Embraced*, which featured stories of women from around the world and their battles and triumphs over the seemingly ubiquitous hatred of our bodies and the desperate need to conform to a slim, white ideal. The documentary was well received and even had a modest but positive effect on those who viewed it and their body image, according to independent research. Brumfitt followed it up with books, speaking engagements and television appearances around the world, in which she encouraged women to love their bodies regardless of whether they fitted the ideal that has been sold to us for years. She created the *Body Image Movement* to showcase women's bodies as 'a vehicle to their dreams' and offers a four-week challenge where users pay $AU 59 to learn how to 'embrace' their bodies.

Megan Jayne Crabbe, known by her social media handle @bodyposipanda, has also gained a huge following with her 'love your body' message. Crabbe's own story included disordered eating and excessive exercise; she now has a body that is healthier and happier, she says. Her debut book, *Body Positive Power*, details her road to recovery and encourages readers to embrace the parts of themselves that society derides. Her social media following continues to grow, with thousands of new followers every month watching a beautiful and curvy Crabbe dance in her underwear or enjoy beach holidays in bikinis that society still tries to tell her she shouldn't wear.

People everywhere and women in particular have been subject to incredible pressure over their bodies, so it's no wonder that these advocates for a kinder attitude have been so welcomed. However, with their popularity has come a barrage of criticism of body positivity, most notably for normalising obesity. Holliday herself has engaged in public battles on social media with people who chastise her for promoting ill-health. Given that our hardline approach to demanding physical perfection has not worked, is there something in this new, more inclusive and compassionate approach? Do we need to give our bodies tough love to keep them healthy or do we need be kinder? And is body positivity as bad for our physical health as skinny or athletic ideals? Body positivity is a natural and probably necessary retaliation to traditional body-shaming, but if it doesn't promote health, is it any better than other crusades, trends or norms?

Beauty in the eye of the beholder: body image

Body image is a term that is thrown around a lot, but what does it really mean? Body image describes our perceptions and attitudes towards our physical appearance. It is a mixture of how we physically see our bodies, how we feel about them and the resulting behaviours. Those times you have looked down at yourself and thought 'big thighs' or 'nice calves' are all part of your body image; your personal perception of what you look like and how you feel about your body. Body image changes over time, so how you feel as a teenager may evolve as you age. It can even change day-to-day as things happen to you to make you feel differently about this wonderful vessel you get around in.

What is interesting, but not at all surprising, is that our own experiences or thoughts are more powerful than other people's opinions of us. Our perceptions are much more prone to being distorted and shaped rather than being an objective or even accurate representation of how things actually are. Our body image changes depending on our mood, whether we've exercised and how we judge ourselves against some ideal or standard. Although others are more objective, what we see in the mirror, distorted or not, is uppermost in our mind. Despite reassurances from our friends, family or partners, we often do not believe them. Our views are much more powerful than anyone else's.

Because most research into body image has come from studying eating disorders, it's had a particular focus on younger women, who were thought to suffer disproportionately. However, research into the origin and effects of body image has now expanded to include people with a disability, those from diverse backgrounds and also men, who have in the past been absent.

Unsurprisingly, the fascination with body image has spread and companies such as Dove and Aerie now use it as a marketing tool, creating campaigns that are designed to make us feel better about ourselves. A study of 200 women looked at how they felt about their bodies after viewing the Aerie campaign and found a small decrease in body dissatisfaction compared with looking at the usual, retouched and slim underwear models. But let's be honest, at the end of the day, these companies need to sell soap and undies too and tapping into the zeitgeist doesn't hurt.

The academic definition of body image looks at many different facets of our attitudes towards and behaviours regarding our body. However, research has shown that body image is strongly aligned with our weight and is seen predominantly as a women's issue. Since body image has been linked to women and eating disorders and our society loves to emphasise weight, this is not surprising. However, body image is a continuum; it is not just about our weight and certainly not something that only women think about.

How we see our bodies develops over our whole lifetime. Children learn from an early age to compare themselves to others; including how their bodies look. Preschoolers learn that society disapproves of fat people, setting them up to have positive and negative views about their bodies and others from very early on. Throughout life, we're exposed to a variety of messages from our family, the media and our peers about what is good and bad about bodies; how we process those messages affects how we see ourselves. Overwhelmingly, those messages show a preference for thin women, muscular men and Caucasians in general; we equate these to health and happiness. It's not uncommon to think that once you look like this ideal, your body image will magically improve. Spoiler alert: it doesn't.

Because of this, the body image we develop can be positive or negative and all the shades of grey in between. I think that the definition of positive body image by researcher Tracy Tylka PhD is beautiful because it truly encompasses all the wonderful things our bodies can do. She says that positive body image is love and respect for the body that allows us to appreciate our own unique beauty, what our body can do for us and to admire our body even if it doesn't fit society's ideal. It enables us to feel comfortable and confident with our body and emphasise its assets, not its imperfections. Positive body image also allows us to disregard the negative information and incorporate the good; what it isn't is an unwavering love for your body, thinking you look banging hot no matter what happens.

When we have preferences for body characteristics that are different to the ones we think we have, this is called body dissatisfaction. We develop these feelings about our body from life experiences, the culture we live in, the people close to us, teasing, our personality type and our beliefs about what bodies should be. All of these lead to behaviours that can perpetuate or even worsen these feelings. As I wrote these two paragraphs, I was saddened to think that I was struggling to think of a woman I know who isn't dissatisfied with her body. And I know many men who share this dissatisfaction too. I've seen many bodies in my career and despite it being in a purely professional setting, the number of people who apologise for their body is sad. (Trust me, you do not need to and you should never do that.)

Scarily, this perception starts early. Between 40 and 50 per cent of six to 12-year-old girls are dissatisfied with their bodies. Six years old! Girls are taught the value of appearance more than boys, with toys promoting beauty over ability. (I'm looking at you, Barbie!) Kids who internalise these messages develop higher levels of body dissatisfaction. The trend continues through their life with 70 per cent of teenage girls wanting to be thinner – far higher than the percentage of girls who are actually overweight. Teenage girls seem to feel that being thinner will result in them being happier, healthier and better-looking and 70 per cent point to the lithe, youthful figures in magazines as 'ideal bodies'.

The more time we spend looking at perfect images, the more we internalise them; here our family and peers have an important role to play. Of course, every culture has differing beauty ideals, but even in non-Caucasian populations, there is conformity. African-American women are strongly influenced by their families and are a little more accepting of larger bodies. Hispanic women are influenced by the media and family, but their curvy natural body type makes it nearly impossible to meet the common standard. Jennifer Lopez has achieved this but she is often quoted in magazines detailing the intense workouts she does or listing all the foods she avoids eating to look the way she does.

Into adult life, we still want to be thinner but then on top of that we want to be younger too. Men also feel the pressure to look a certain way, with the current body ideal emphasising 'ripped' and muscular. As we know, very few of the ideals sold to us have anything to do with health. In fact, in order to come close to meeting these impossible standards, a lot of us need to sacrifice our health and use dangerous methods to get there.

Take those muscular men for example. The pictures may conveniently fail to show their dangerous abuse of anabolic steroids in order to achieve the shredded, muscular ideal. Fashion models, the long-standing body ideal for women, have been frequently associated with unhealthy eating such as extreme calorie restriction and dangerous exercise levels. Add in the posing, lighting and editing and we have no idea what we're looking at, even though we think their physique holds the answer to our physical and mental betterment.

The dangers of weight bias

As we are sold and internalise this idea of what an ideal body should be, a phenomenon called weight bias develops. Weight bias is a preference for slimmer bodies and negative attitudes towards bigger bodies. Weight bias leads to all kinds of negative consequences, including discrimination at work, in education and in healthcare. It's perpetuated by the media and can also have negative effects on our relationships.

The sad thing is that we can all internalise this weight bias and direct it at our own bodies. Weight bias internalisation is related to body dissatisfaction but is a little different. It is when we take on board and believe these negative messages about weight. This isn't just something bigger people do; a huge proportion of us internalise that thin is better and direct that towards ourselves in terms of what we think about our bodies and what we do to avoid gaining weight. Sometimes, this internalised stereotype about weight leads us to see our own bodies in a negative and critical light, altering our body image – this can result in us doing things that are not good for our physical or mental health. Cast your mind back to the conversations you have had with yourself or people around you, just in the last week. How much of that talk was about the very many problems you perceive about your own body? Fat talk is a pretty common topic of conversation and involves mutually sharing the things about your appearance that you don't like. Fat talk, very common amongst women, has been associated with body image problems, depression and disordered eating. It's yet another way we perpetuate a hatred for our bodies and it has real mental and physical consequences. It might make you feel like you're not alone for a few minutes, but fat talk is a crappy way of relating to other people or making yourself feel better. It does the exact opposite and should be avoided at all costs.

It's fairly obvious that all this judgement of ourselves and others is bad for our mental health. Weight bias internalisation, body dissatisfaction and body image problems are associated with depression, anxiety and low self-esteem.

Weight bias in particular is seen in the way people seek out healthcare and their subsequent treatment by health-care professionals. People who have a higher BMI are less likely to seek healthcare when they need it for fear of stigma or unwanted conversations about their weight. Obese people who see a doctor for a non-weight related problem are more likely to have their weight brought up in conversation or have screening done for complications of their weight. Now; as a doctor, I find this challenging because every time we see someone, it's an opportunity to catch illness early or help people prevent it altogether.

However, when it's unwanted or delivered in the wrong way, even if it's well-meaning, it might have the opposite effect.

Health-care workers need to learn what to say, as well as how to say it, and prioritise health over weight loss. We need to understand that words can hurt; decades of fat bias have permeated every aspect of people's lives and it's not making anyone healthier.

Even something as vital as a breast self-examination is affected by our perceptions. Women who are dissatisfied with their breasts are less likely to do a self-exam, which can be vital to detect breast cancer early – and early detection saves lives.

Outside the doctor's office is really where health is cultivated, in the behaviours we undertake to keep ourselves healthy. Having body image or body dissatisfaction issues can have a profound negative effect on whether we exercise or eat well. Trying to shame someone into being healthy truly doesn't work – shame is more likely to result in behaviours such as binge eating. Adolescents who *think* they are overweight, whether they are or not, are more likely to do things that increase the risk for obesity, such as not exercising and eating unhealthy foods.

Looking at the effects of weight bias reveals that weight discrimination actually increases mortality. The reason for this is unclear but could relate to engaging in unhealthy behaviours or avoiding the doctor due to shame or embarrassment. Basically, thinking or knowing that you're unhealthy doesn't always help and could even cause harm.

On the other hand, having a positive body image seems to improve both mental and physical health. Positive body image seems to be associated with less depression, better self-esteem, less dieting and even doing simple things like protecting your skin from the sun, a vital part of avoiding skin cancer. Being able to appreciate the good things about your body or, even better, focusing on its abilities and not its appearance means you tend to exercise and eat good food, avoiding diets and bingeing. Kindness and compassion to ourselves is actually the key.

Body positivity: a hero for our time?

If body dissatisfaction and weight bias is the villain of this story, then body positivity claims to be our hero. Body positivity has sprung up in recent years, partly as an offshoot of the fat acceptance movement, which aims to reduce many forms of stigma directed against people with obesity, from society at large to the medical profession. While 'fat acceptance' is a movement purely for people with obesity (one which has been met with significant scepticism), body positivity aims to be more inclusive and more conducive to overall health and wellbeing. In the online sphere body positivity, or as it's often called on social media, BoPo, has amassed a huge following with role models such as the aforementioned Tess Holliday, Taryn Brumfitt and Megan Jayne Crabbe having millions of followers between them. The body positivity hashtag is used in millions of online posts on a wide variety of pictures.

Body positivity is more about developing positive body image by cultivating acceptance and appreciation of all bodies, not just those that are overweight or obese. Fat acceptance is narrowly defined and has the backing of organisations like the National Association to Advance Fat Acceptance, while body positivity has a much wider reach. Body positivity was coined around the early-to-mid 1990s to fight eating disorders. It has evolved but at its heart is a pushback against negative body image and the vast cultural, financial and even medical ways in which we criticise our bodies.

What's the difference between body positivity and positive body image?

It's important to understand that body positivity is not positive body image. Body positivity is more of a social justice movement, thanks in large to its roots in fat acceptance and the drive to normalise how society sees and treats all kinds of bodies. Positive body image is how we see ourselves in that positive, compassionate yet realistic light with a degree of resilience. It's an individual thing, while body positivity is for everyone and especially for those who have previously been excluded.

This movement directly opposes the thin, fit, white ideal as being the only way to look and all of the messages and industries that sell us this notion.

Alongside body positivity and fat acceptance, the Health at Every Size (HAES) philosophy has gained in popularity. Although its roots extend further back to the 1960s, the HAES term is also closely related to fat acceptance and has evolved from being relatively underground to a popular diet-adverse movement. It is now a health approach with some science behind it. HAES exists to promote self-care predominantly by encouraging healthy behaviours while stringently avoiding weight bias and being wholly inclusive of all bodies. HAES does not have anything to do with weight loss; in fact it actively avoids promoting it. When we take weight out of the equation and focus on health, research has shown some promising results. When followed for two years, a group of women taking the HAES approach of ignoring weight showed improvements in measures of health, both physically and mentally.

Given that negative body image and body dissatisfaction are associated with all of these adverse outcomes and weight stigma causes enormous amounts of harm, it's reasonable to expect that body positivity is our hero. It's a way to fight against glossy magazines telling us not to eat a certain food or the latest round of skinny Instagram darlings showing us the bodies we ought to want and giving us the unscientific and unhealthy tools to get there.

Either as a society or as health professionals, we have a history of doing a really bad job of helping people with a lifestyle disease. Rather than lending a helping hand to those who need it, we shame them. We attack rather than support and that bias has created generations of utterly miserable people who hate their bodies and suffer the resulting poor health. It's really no wonder then that body positivity, fat acceptance and Health at Every Size have become part of the zeitgeist as well as a tool in the health-care professional's armament.

Whether you are underweight, overweight or somewhere inbetween, problems with body image harm us all and just keep perpetuating the ideal that being skinny will bring you health and happiness. That kind of thinking probably doesn't even bring you skinny and it certainly doesn't bring you happiness. Body positivity and any other movement aimed at destroying stigma are a necessary and important part of our evolution towards finding a better way to promote health and ignore the harmful messages we've been sent for many years.

Is it really good for us?

Scrolling through the Instagram posts of people like Tess Holliday and Megan Jayne Crabbe reveals an enormous amount of goodwill towards the celebration of them as positive role models. But it also uncovers a whole host of people calling them fat and other names because they don't find them attractive. There is also another group of people who are commenting on these photos, expressing concern for their physical health. In return, Holliday and Crabbe often post back that they are healthy and are simply choosing to live a life that suits them and makes them happy. These so-called 'concern trolls' are expressing concern for the women's weight – but it's just another way of saying they hate fat people. Every time Holliday pops up in the media, UK commentator Piers Morgan is never far behind, expressing his concern for (or perhaps disgust at) her in a manner that is condescending and belittling.

It's not just body positive influencers such as these women who are touting the 'everyone can be healthy' tagline. A growing number of health-care professionals, including dietitians, are extolling the virtues of this philosophy. They share information on why dieting is bad, obesity is not as bad as we thought and that trying to lose weight is pointless or shameful. This is probably a way of buying into the multi-billion-dollar industries that want us to be healthy but in fact just want our money. These experts share academic articles on how BMI has been debunked (partially true) and how obesity isn't associated with a particular disease (not entirely true) and argue with online followers as much as the more prolific body positive role models when their ideals are challenged.

The data doesn't always hold strong either. Body positivity or Health at Every Size health-care professionals are just as prone to posting data that suits their cause. Some cite 20-year-old scientific studies that have been better defined or challenged by more recent and credible science. Some post articles on how obesity is actually good in some circumstances, quietly ignoring the large volume of science that opposes this finding. I feel like everyone is not looking at the broader picture and is just choosing sides. One side says, hands down, being fat is bad and you must lose weight above all else. The other side says fat people are only sick because of the bias they experience. It's far too simplistic a way of looking at health. The middle ground, where obesity is a complex illness that can have complications for some people in certain circumstances and that bias, stigma and traditional dieting approaches are not very helpful, seems to elude both sides of the debate. We're at war with each other and being forced to pick sides, when the reality is that there is no black and white, just shades of grey where we could meet and truly make a difference to people's health.

Body positivity has also come under fire for its lack of inclusivity. While it arguably does a better job than the diet brigade, body positivity still tends to show women who are not so far from the accepted norm. There is still a tendency to focus on women who are white and traditionally beautiful and are simply acknowledging their relaxed stomachs rather than being a genuine challenge to the norm. Actor and activist Jameela Jamil is an outspoken critic of beauty norms and diets and yet she herself receives huge amounts of criticism for daring to have such an opinion because she's deemed to be slim and beautiful and extremely privileged. I think it's safe to say that she knows that. It's definitely important to call out body positive activists who aren't inclusive but you seem damned either way. Say something and you're too slim/beautiful to be allowed an opinion, say nothing and you're complicit/ empowering the patriarchy/not checking your privilege. It's a complex world out there.

Body positivity at its core is there to accept everyone, yet it often falls into the traps that plague other movements. It is so frequently associated with showing bodies that are bigger that it forgets to show bodies that are disabled, of different ethnicities, have stomas and scars or any one of the other myriad forms our bodies come in. We are, once again, so focused on fatness versus thinness that we forget all these other people whose bodies don't fit the norm. They are often looking at their bodies in a different way and focusing instead on what they can achieve.

All social movements are at risk of commodification and body positivity is no different. Body positive models have been seen to promote the same things they want to derail, including those 'flat tummy teas'. This goes a long way to undermining the ethos of the body positive movement and is more in keeping with the sort of marketing we see from the diet industries.

Brands, of course, get in on the action where there is money to be made. While it's important that plus-sized clothing exists so that people who are outside the traditional sizes can enjoy shopping, there is a commercial motive. Personal care brand Dove was an early adopter of body positive campaigns, showing women wearing no make-up, underwear-clad women of all shapes and sizes, and women having a stranger describe how beautiful they are. However, research has shown that the promotion of plus-size bodies in this context doesn't necessarily change the level of heavy self-criticism, referred to as body-policing. The Dove campaigns have been generally well received by consumers but when brands post images purporting to be 'body positive', but featuring only slender white models, consumers are quick to react.

While the move away from heavily airbrushed marketing featuring young and seemingly flawless models is a positive direction, research suggests that this kind of marketing has only a small effect on body positivity. In addition, socially sensitive marketing simply allows brands that are selling cosmetics, clothing and other lifestyle paraphernalia to tap into a new market, while still selling products that body-positive warriors find objectionable. The brands appear better, more trustworthy and healthier because of their new association, when the reality is that they are still selling beauty.

Is it all an excuse?

The biggest criticism of all these movements comes in the form of health concerns. Whether they are directed at the body positive idol or society at large, many people fear that body positivity promotes obesity and excuses behaviours that stop people becoming or staying healthy. Since our society is sinking huge amounts of time and money into fighting non-communicable diseases, it seems counterproductive or even dangerous for these kinds of messages to circulate.

The more we see people who are larger, the more we are likely to normalise these bodies, according to research. A UK study found that a high number of people who were overweight or obese perceived their weight as 'about right'. This study has been criticised for not looking at actual health measures or referencing the large number of studies that show telling people they're overweight doesn't translate into meaningful weight loss. It also ignores the fact that stigma is damaging to people and normalising different bodies is desperately needed. Labelling children as big seems to correlate with weight gain throughout their life and a large-scale study from Korea actually showed physical health is threatened just by thinking you're overweight, regardless of whether you are or not. It will be interesting to see how this translates to health behaviours because that's where our focus should be – what we do, not what we look like. Let's be honest though, knowing we're fat won't make us thin. And thinking fat is okay won't make us fat – most of us are still petrified of getting out of shape either because our clothes won't fit or we won't be attractive. Seeing Tess Holliday is not going to make you gain tens of kilos, just as watching a Victoria's Secret show won't make you lose tens of kilos. Normalising bigger or different-looking bodies is not the worst thing in the world. Rather than categorising bodies, let's just begin to understand that we come in all kinds of shapes, sizes, colours or abilities and work with what we have.

That doesn't let body positivity or Health at Every Size completely off the hook. While most experts agree that we need to adopt a different approach, free of stigma, commercialisation and junk science, they also question the blind following of these schools of thought. We say that people can be healthy at every size, fit and fat, or immune to the ill effects of bad behaviours but the reality just doesn't support this. Even if we acknowledge that some people who smoke or drink to excess will still live long and healthy lives, they are statistically the exception rather than the rule. The link between obesity and heart disease is incredibly strong, so to say that you can be healthy at any size, especially over the longer term, isn't telling the whole story.

Once you have gained enough weight to be considered overweight or obese and to have developed complications, the weight is hard, if not impossible, to shift. Then there are issues about endless weight cycling and how that can also result in illness. Critics of the HAES or body positivity approach say that by normalising being overweight, people might avoid trying to lose weight and consequently suffer these ill effects. It may even stop people from investing in prevention, which is better than a cure.

Some body positive advocates have shared posts on social media criticising women who share their body transformations and weight loss progress, especially if that person has a public presence. Australian radio host Mel Grieg copped this treatment and came out swinging, saying she wouldn't be shamed for sharing her health journey. Her lifestyle had been very unhealthy and she shouldn't have been discouraged from wanting to lose weight and quit bad habits, including drinking too much alcohol. Plus-size model Ashley Graham received comments from ardent followers denouncing her when she lost weight, saying that she was betraying body positivity. Body positivity and wanting to lose weight can co-exist, but there are noisy zealots on both sides of this debate.

Peta Adams and Tyson Tripcony are Australian dietitians who run Dietitian Life, a website and social media platform dedicated to supporting dietitians. They and their professional clients are quite vocal about the drawbacks of the HAES paradigm and have found themselves in the middle of a vicious war. Adams and Tripcony say that the movement is poorly named as you cannot be healthy at *every* size. You can be *healthier* at every size, they say, and they are highly critical of the way the science of weight is ignored in favour of loving your body. 'We have clients who have joint pain related to their weight, but as long as they're positive about their bones, that pain will just go away?' they query. They believe that shaming people, forcing them to pick sides and ignoring the science is just as impractical as our current flawed approach. I agree; we can't wholly ignore the science. HAES has an unfortunate name because we can be healthier whatever our size; just because the wellness industry has some serious limitations doesn't mean we should bag out everyone who wants to eat well, lose weight and feel better.

Body balance

If we are to hold body positive role models up to the same scrutiny as those peddling diets and exercise regimens, the same rules apply. If we say that the attractive, toned and lean bodies we see on social media and in magazines aren't telling us the whole truth about their health practices, then we can say the same for those on the other team. When body positive role models say they're healthy we take it at face value, as we do for the skinny role models. Are they, though? And, more importantly, is it any of our business? No, it's not. Your own health is your business and moralising your concern over someone else's health is unnecessary. However, we do know from science that just saying you're healthy because you don't have any problems isn't the whole story; you may be okay now, but you could be sick in the future. Saying you're fit but fat can be misleading since a number of people who are overweight or obese are likely to go on to develop heart disease or diabetes if we follow them for ten years or even longer. Either way, stop staring at the fat rolls or the abs on the Instagram photo because it's misleading.

What probably matters most are the things you can't see: what you do to be healthy and what we can measure about your health, not a filtered photograph.

You can be healthy or healthier whatever your body size or bad habits, but this information is often absent from some of the body positive content. This is a missed opportunity. To see some of these body positive idols exercise and eat nutritious food, both of which can vastly improve your health irrespective of size, would be a much better middle ground. Our idols should holistically promote a better ideal, not just campaign that you don't have to look like a Victoria's Secret model to be photographed in your knickers. We're letting the tribal nature of the debate interfere with our ability to see another side of the story and come to a safe and healthy reality.

'Love yourself, embrace yourself' is what we're told from the body positive tribe, as if this were enough to erase decades of deeply ingrained ideas and dissatisfaction. Whether it's through books, social media or training courses designed to help you love your body, this approach is far too simplistic and has been criticised by experienced psychologists and body image disorder experts. People tend to struggle with the kind of turnaround that is self-led and supposedly as easy as touching the tummy you hate or saying affirmations in a mirror. Years of psychological conditioning can be challenging to untangle. Truly loving your body could be yet another daily chore that is bound to fail. Changing the way you think in this environment is just as hard as trying to eat vegetables inside a fast food store. It's a simplistic notion that doesn't address all of the problems around body image and sets us up to fail at something yet again.

If negative body image and all that it generates is the enemy, body positivity is a flawed hero. Promoting health and fitness with photos of tiny waists and beautiful bikinis, and body positivity with tummy rolls and cake-eating, are two sides of the same coin. Body positivity doesn't directly promote obesity, just as looking at a picture of a fitness model doesn't give everyone an eating disorder; it's just not that simple. Health is not about size but when size has an impact on health, it has to be acknowledged. Neither side of this debate can ignore the science at hand. We can fight bias and disease at the same time, so long as we do it with compassion and without judgement, united for a good, science-based outcome.

Body positivity and all of its close relatives, Health at Every Size and even fat acceptance have something important to bring to the quest for health, just as some people promoting healthy eating and exercise do. The simple fact is that you can't shame someone into being healthy; shame and discrimination have the opposite effect. Body positivity can be a vital part of our quest for health by helping to remove the stigma we all carry. Body positivity might be able to counter the moral failure we associate with being overweight and allow us to stop equating people's appearance with their character and health. Both these estimations are misleading. This does not ignore the fact that body positivity has shortcomings, like any field. By ignoring the very real health problems we all face, it's missing a great opportunity to shape us to be healthier and live a life in which we are not judged for our appearance.

Body positivity does not promote obesity. Our society has a dreadful body image overall and this is doing far more damage to our health than Holliday, Crabbe or any other curvy woman. We must stop placing so much emphasis on matching our appearance to an unachievable ideal and start to focus instead on the uniqueness and capability of our bodies. Decades of hating our bodies hasn't worked, so loving them may well be the way forward. Body positivity has flaws, but that doesn't mean that it's entirely wrong; the truth lies somewhere in between. As the research evolves and our knowledge increases, it would be good to get a new paradigm where everyone becomes more mindful of the effects, both good and bad, of being body positive.

Self-compassion: a science-based answer

Body positivity is trying to teach us is to love ourselves, despite the fact we've been conditioned to do the opposite, with the aim of improving our health. It is an important change that needs to happen. We cannot deny the powerful impact that stigma, body dissatisfaction and weight bias has on our wellbeing, just as we cannot deny the detrimental effects of obesity, inactivity and a low-nutrition diet. If body positivity is not the perfect answer, is there anything that is?

Self-compassion is a psychological phenomenon that was suggested to me by multiple experts as an important psychological tool for maintaining health, both mental and physical. Self-compassion is the ability to be compassionate towards yourself when you think you're inadequate or have failed. There are three components to it; self-kindness, common humanity and mindfulness. Self-kindness means that you are kind to yourself rather than reaching for that familiar collection of self-criticisms. Part of this common humanity is remembering that failure and bumps in the road are a normal part of our existence. It's comforting to know that we're not alone. And of course, mindfulness, a hot topic at the moment, is all about acknowledging your situation and your feelings without dwelling on them or becoming judgemental. When we are motivated by self-criticism, it does not sustain our goals in the long run, but self-compassion can do that.

Far from being a way to let yourself off the hook, self-compassion gives you the tools to dust yourself off, acknowledge the problem and move forward. It's realistic and leads to achieving peace of mind. Rather than saying 'screw it' and giving up or berating yourself, self-compassion allows you to see failure as a point of growth and improvement. I find that the things we say to ourselves for a dietary slip-up or missing a run are overly critical. We come down on ourselves so hard and yet, very few of us would take the same approach to a friend. We say to our reflection in the mirror that we look so fat and yet, we would reassure a friend that they look great or offer them love and unconditional support to eat better. We would join them on long walks at the weekend to help motivate them, yet we never afford ourselves that same kindness. Self-compassion is about taking those kind actions and turning them inwards for ourselves.

Research has shown that self-compassion can significantly improve body image and body dissatisfaction. It can also be learnt. What fascinates me is that the benefits aren't just psychological but also physical. Generally, having self-compassion can lead to healthy behaviours like exercising and eating well. It has even been shown to help people quit smoking more quickly than if they are hypercritical of their efforts. Even in people with diabetes, learning self-compassion allowed them to feel less distressed about their condition and even resulted in better control of their blood sugars. This is an important finding and a real testament to the power of our emotions.

Self-compassion is not tough love, nor is it blind. Self-compassion is a much more realistic and science-based way of improving our health and wellbeing. To me, self-compassion is more like saying to yourself: 'Well, I skipped that workout; but that's okay – it happens and I'm going to make it up later or try to avoid missing it again in the future.' It's not the self-berating response where missing one workout leads to a food binge or punishing yourself with a run twice as long. Self-compassion is the self-love body positive champions want us to have, but in a way that is realistic and scientific and leads to improvement without self-criticism.

Chapter 8

EXTRAORDINARY BODIES

'What's your excuse?'

**MARIA KANG,
3 MONTHS AFTER GIVING BIRTH TO HER THIRD CHILD**

Would it surprise you to know that the vast majority of medical research is done on men? Probably not. Men are great subjects, to be honest, in large part because of their lack of pregnancy. It's hard to test a drug on a woman who is or might be pregnant or allow for those crazy oestrogen effects that can muddy the waters of our carefully designed clinical trials. There is one notable exception in the world of health-related research and it's nothing to do with babies. Research into body image, eating disorders, social media and the impact they have on our health is largely done on women. Young, white, educated, slim, cis-gendered, able-bodied, heterosexual women. This means that anyone who looks, acts or was born another way is vastly under-represented when we try to unravel all of the issues around health and wellness. Not to let the gender bias in medical research off the hook; this is probably one of the few places in scientific literature where women do actually come out on top.

Not every body is the same though. Neither is everyone's experience of what constitutes health or illness or what you're willing to put yourself through in order to be healthier, happier, slimmer or more beautiful. The fit/slim/beautiful-equals-healthy ideal is hard enough for those of us who at least share some of the same characteristics of those we're supposed to idolise, but can you imagine how hard it must be if you're not even close to that? Imagine how hard it must be if you are not able-bodied, have scars or have survived a serious illness. Imagine if you're too busy growing a human inside you or you're male or somewhere else on the continuum of humanness. That has not stopped the immense pressure to conform to a healthy ideal, to act or look a certain way. It does not offer immunity from judgement, internal or external, and it certainly does not offer immunity from harm.

Some time ago I met a woman who was a patient on my ward. She was born with a condition of her heart that was a constant threat to her life. To fix this, she faced major heart surgery. She sticks in my mind for two major reasons: firstly, her surgery was one of the most stressful and complicated I had experienced in my career and during the first few hours afterwards she wasn't expected to make it through the night. The second reason was really fascinating. Months after the surgery, I examined her body, which was covered in scars and disfigurements. I listened to her heart and lungs and remarked how well she was doing. After all, it felt like just yesterday that she had seemed to be heading towards the light. I asked her straight how she felt about her broken body, which was irrevocably changed, covered in bandages and plastic tubes. With immaculate hair, stylish glasses and a thin veil of make-up, she said to me straightaway: 'How can I not love my body? It survived.' It brought tears to my eyes. Here was a woman who faced death because of her body's medical issues and yet she admired it so much. I think I was moved by her openness and bravery but also by the guilt I felt; I don't know if I have that much admiration for myself. I'm not sure that many people do.

That conversation got me wondering about how those who have a difference, ranging from the everyday occurrence of pregnancy to the unexpected, such as a serious illness or an amputation, fit into a world where beauty is a surrogate for health. Into a world that says health is a specific and fashionable workout that you do or the diet that you consume. What if you can't do these things? What if, by virtue of your difference, the world expects twice as much of you, as they do a pregnant woman or a new mother? How do you feel about your body and how do you define its health and wellbeing after losing a part of it or gaining a part of another? The wellness industry is so geared towards pushing the 'norm' and yet it still tries to exert its influence on those who have less chance of meeting its unrealistic expectations.

Boobs rule

Breasts are fascinating organs. Along with being responsible for the very physiological process of feeding a child, they are there for arousal and even define a woman's own femininity and sexuality. Given the expectations around breasts, it's no wonder that breast cancer is at the forefront of many people's minds. Breast cancer is the most common form of cancer in women. However, the most common form of cancer death in women is from lung cancer. Breast cancer awareness has done the most magnificent job of changing the way we look for and treat the disease, with five-year survival rates in developed countries well over 80 per cent. Very few other cancers can claim to have made such significant inroads in this kind of treatment. Buoyed by celebrites who have been open about breast cancer, such as Angelina Jolie, this disease has a remarkable presence in our minds and this awareness results in early detection.

In cancer, early detection reigns supreme. Whatever the type of cancer, the earlier it is detected, the sooner it can be treated and the chances of survival are greatly increased. For some cancers, by the time symptoms appear, the disease has progressed; so the introduction of screening programs dedicated to picking up cancers before symptoms show leads to less death from that cancer and a better quality of life. Breast cancer screening has been a great success; it starts with a breast self-exam and enlists your local doctor or a mammogram program to try to catch it early.

Body image can be an important predictor in women's health behaviours. Body image problems are related to a number of things that hinder rather than help our health, including substance abuse, inappropriate or inadequate exercise, poor disease management, tanning or risky sexual behaviour. It's also possible that poor body image could reduce the rate at which women screen for various cancers. Women are encouraged to undergo screening for breast, cervical and skin cancers from a relatively early age but it is a very intimate process. Screening yourself involves a level of touching and familiarity as well as curiosity about and perhaps comfort with your own body. Having screening done by a health-care professional means you are usually partly naked and bearing your most intimate body parts to someone else. It is confronting and uncomfortable.

For breast cancer, most recommendations say that a woman should perform a monthly breast self-examination from the time she's 20. When a woman is over 50 years old, she has mammograms every two years. Research has shown that fewer than one third of women regularly perform their monthly self-exam and only 27 per cent perform them adequately. Some of this relates to education, anxiety over finding something wrong or not knowing how to do a breast exam properly; one factor that has been explored is BMI. The science has shown that the more underweight or overweight someone is, the *less* likely they are to undergo the various health checks they need, especially in white women.

Now, there are a multitude of reasons this might be true, such as weight stigma or socio-economic status. However, body image could also have a role to play. A number of research projects have found that the higher someone's body dissatisfaction is, the less likely they are to have these screening exams, even those they do themselves. Even just focusing on breasts alone, feeling dissatisfied with your breasts, either their size or overall appearance, seems to lead to having fewer mammograms and less self-examination. Let's be clear here; screening for cancer absolutely saves lives. Yet, we live in a society that has allowed us to cultivate such negative views of our own bodies that we forego, or are maybe too afraid or ashamed to attend, lifesaving exams or tests. What a messed-up world we live in.

I chatted about this over dinner with a group of friends, all doctors. What started off as a conversation about how much everyone hates pap smears or doesn't do breast exams as often as they should (most of the time they forgot) quickly evolved into a discussion about how much everyone hates getting naked in front of someone else. They said they always wondered what the doctor was thinking about their bikini wax or breast size. One woman said that she was putting off getting her annual skin check until she had lost some weight. She said the last time she saw her dermatologist she was about 10 kilograms lighter and would be horrified to have him look at her stomach until it had shrunk. And then we all realised what we were saying. As doctors, we had examined bodies of every shape, size, colour and even smell. And you know what? We were professional. Yet we were embarrassed at how someone else might judge the attractiveness of our bodies in the course of life-saving medical care; so much so that it affected whether or not we had it.

(Interestingly, putting a focus on appearance with the ageing effects of sun exposure seems to increase the use of sun protection. It seems caring about your looks can, in that instance, make you healthier. Professor Diana Harcourt from the University of Western England's Centre for Appearance Research is cautious about tapping into this aspect. She says that although appearance could be a way of deterring people from smoking, for instance, it may also increase negative views of ageing and lead people to engage in cosmetic surgery or other treatments to stay looking young. Many of these carry risks of their own to our health.)

Around 40 per cent of breast cancers are detected by self-examination and nearly 60 per cent by mammogram. For those who go on to have a diagnosis of breast cancer, the treatment depends on the type of cancer and how advanced it is. For most people, it involves one or a combination of surgery, chemotherapy, radiotherapy and hormonal or immunotherapy. The increased survival rates are a great advance, but they also mean women are living longer with the consequences of treatment. Obviously, cancer can be a life-threatening disease but it can also be very visible. The side effects of treatment can include scarring, weight changes, hair loss, lymphedema and the symptoms of menopause. These changes can result in body image concerns; up to 77 per cent have long-lasting concerns.

It's easy to dismiss this as frivolous, given the fact that the treatment is a means to a very important end. But for many women, breasts are an important part of defining their femininity. Breast cancer treatment might involve wearing different clothes, a prosthesis or a head scarf or wig. What may be a very private issue becomes public because of the overtly physical nature of changes, such as hair loss, lack of breasts or scars. However, feeling good about yourself during and after cancer treatment is important for both psychological and physical health. Poor body image after breast cancer treatment leads to anxiety, depression and less intimacy with a partner. A large meta-analysis of body image and breast cancer showed that younger breast-cancer patients may have more body image concerns which can lead to more pain, more breast dissatisfaction and more reconstructive and cosmetic procedures. Every medical procedure carries risks so this dissatisfaction should not be taken lightly and it may be associated with lower survival rates. This link is not supported by strong evidence – just one study done a number of years ago – so should be looked at cautiously. That being said, we do see worse physical health outcomes in lots of diseases, including cancer and heart disease, in people with anxiety and depression or low social support, so how we feel in ourselves and with other people may have an impact.

Not everyone who has breast cancer treatment will develop poor body image; it's a little difficult to predict who will have difficulties. Some women see changes to their body as just a matter of course in their treatment, while others are deeply affected. It doesn't seem to be reliably predicted by age or gender (men get breast cancer too) but one factor could be how someone felt about their appearance before their diagnosis. One interesting aspect is that women who are undergoing or have finished breast cancer treatment seem to be more susceptible to the beauty ideals perpetrated by social media and the mainstream media. Their illness and their treatment pushes them further and further away from what we're told is beautiful and this can contribute to their poor body image. So, our society makes women with cancer feel even worse.

In cancer-related programs such as Look Good, Feel Better, people on treatment get pampered and learn how to use make-up and wigs to help them feel more attractive. These programs are generally well-received by patients but don't always show long-term results on body image. That's not to say they aren't useful; in fact, they're a tremendous addition to the growing stable of cancer treatments which encompass making the whole person feel better, not just fighting the disease. A recent pilot study from the Centre for Appearance Research showed some promising results for a psychological intervention that really got to the core of body image concerns around breast cancer treatment and body image in general. In the pilot program, women received support and counselling over seven weeks, led by a clinical psychologist and a peer; someone who had been through the same process. They were taught how to identify unhelpful thoughts, how to take care of their body image and how to be aware of the thin–youthful ideal. Results published in *Body Image* journal showed improved body satisfaction for its participants, which was important for their mental wellbeing. We will need to wait to see if these kinds of interventions improve the physical and mental health of all cancer patients but so far, it's very hopeful.

In an effort to regain some normality, a number of women who have had breast cancer will choose to have a reconstructive procedure. In my days as a plastic surgery registrar, I used to see many women who had undergone a mastectomy and then faced major surgery to restore their body. There are many different surgical options available, but they're not all suitable for all women. They range from implants to borrowing muscles from the back or the abdomen to re-create a breast, even a nipple. It's an important part of the treatment process for a number of women – it allows them to feel more 'normal' or feminine or be intimate with their partner again. Interestingly though, women with poorer body image tend to be the least satisfied with the reconstructive results and more likely to undergo repeat surgical procedures, despite having an objectively good reconstruction. Researchers believe that this has a lot to do with unrealistic expectations. If we're pursuing surgery to fix a problem that isn't wholly physical, it seems the risks may well outweigh any benefits.

The way body image affects both detecting and treating breast cancer made me wonder how our society's demands for a perfect body and, specifically, perfect breasts, actually create body image problems. Unfortunately, it's hard to say, although being appearance focused can leave us wide open to feeling the sting of anything that changes it. Professor Harcourt says that, although appearance may seem trivial to some, it's an important way someone with a serious illness can gain back control over their situation. It's also important not to trivialise the importance of what we look like to our sense of self and wellbeing. For someone with a serious illness or some sort of noticeable physical difference, this is much more than being beautiful. This can be about looking like yourself, being 'normal' or more 'acceptable' to society.

The focus on what you look like when you have a life-threatening disease may seem insignificant to some, but it definitely is not and it's important that we are mindful of that. It's important as a friend or support person to help someone take care of their appearance and address these issues which are much more than skin deep. It may be a time where genuinely trying to look more attractive can improve your health and wellbeing.

Just had a baby? That's no excuse

American personal trainer Maria Kang rose to infamy in 2013 when a photo of her, tiny and taut with three very young children, went viral. Her youngest was only a few months old at the time. She flexed and smiled in a crop top and shorts with the caption over the picture-perfect tableau of her life asking: 'What's your excuse?' Kang was called out by huge numbers of people who accused her of being a bully and a narcissist. It was a great marketing exercise for her business, 'No Excuses Mom', a fitness program that provided both free workouts in the local community but also the obligatory DVDs and books that any aspiring fitness empire-maker sells as a matter of course. Kang is not the first nor the last person to place pressure on pregnant women or new mothers to look and act a certain way. Whether the latest celebrity has 'bounced back' from having a baby is regular fodder for women's magazines and social media. Actor Kate Hudson has even signed on to be the newest face of Weight Watchers (aka WW in its attempt at being modern and inclusive). This move angered many given that Hudson is by most standards a healthy, even slim, weight, plus she has more resources to stay slim than your average weight-watcher. The Duchess of Cambridge has also snapped back into shape three times and, even though she stood on the steps of the Lindo Wing three times with a 'mummy tummy' hours after giving birth, she still had perfect blow-dried hair, a full face of make-up, heels and a designer dress.

Even before the baby arrives, a pregnant woman's body is public domain. One of the first lessons I learnt during the medical school obstetrics rotation was not to touch a pregnant woman's stomach without asking; she is not a petting zoo for the public. Even if we're not going around touching women's bodies uninvited, our society seems to feel anyone can have input into what a pregnant mother should and should not do, under the guise of caring about her health and, even better, the baby's. Women are told by anyone who feels the need to share, what to eat, what not to eat, whether or not they should exercise, and how much weight is an appropriate amount to gain during her pregnancy. Alcohol is a particularly sore point for some people; official recommendations say it's safest not to drink because we don't know the safe level. If a woman has a sip of something while pregnant, all hell can break loose.

Pregnancy and motherhood, an intimate and happy time for a lot of people, can lead to a woman's body becoming the subject of everybody's gaze which can create huge amounts of stress for her. Some women feel this pressure because of how differently their body functions and looks, and it can also come from friends and family and, of course, the media. The worry is that the pressure, a lot of which is unrealistic, can lead to body dissatisfaction. A higher BMI and more retention of weight has been associated with feeling worse about your baby body. Some research has also shown a link between body dissatisfaction and depression, disordered eating, less intimacy and shorter duration of breastfeeding. Other studies have even shown that feeling negative about your appearance could even prevent breastfeeding altogether. It might also mean that mothers are less likely to engage in healthy behaviours such as eating well and exercising. In the pressure to bounce back and be 'healthy', we've managed to cultivate a situation where mothers not only feel worse, but it could possibly hamper the health of both mum and baby.

Women tend not to exercise enough during pregnancy; most research suggests that fewer than two in three women get enough exercise at this time. It's actually quite hard to discover how many women might be engaging in diets and exercise programs after having children. Most research on body image and diet or exercise focuses heavily on pregnancy, the really early post-partum period and, of course, how to lose the baby weight. Gaining more weight in pregnancy seems to predict hanging onto it for longer and body image concerns seem to be very prevalent amongst those who can't lose all their body weight. How supportive a woman's environment is, together with her socioeconomic status and what her partner does, is also important. A woman with a healthy partner is often able to exercise or diet more or even quit smoking. Essentially, we know that it's good to be healthy but that's about all we know. Research doesn't tell us how many women fall for the 'you too can snap back like a Victoria's Secret angel' but it does seem to indicate that this sentiment is very harmful.

Weight stigma is known to be problematic for physical and emotional health among the general population but the pressure we're placing on women's weight during pregnancy is a particular problem. In a study of 214 women, researchers looked at the effects of weight stigma on mothers during pregnancy and a year after birth. They found that weight stigma was associated with more weight gain, less weight loss and more post-partum depression. Interestingly, there was no association with blood pressure or cortisol (our major stress hormone). However, pushing women to stay slim during pregnancy and after the birth actually backfires and is not the right way to facilitate their health.

Pregnancy and post-partum, after the baby arrives, is both an incredible and disruptive time. It's also a period when the health of the mother and her baby are very important. During pregnancy, women are monitored with a host of health checks and are given important advice about healthy diets, keeping active and being on the lookout for medical conditions such as gestational diabetes. After the baby is born, the focus does tend to shift a little away from mum and towards the baby. It's something that we have noticed in the realm of heart disease. Pregnancy conditions such as gestational diabetes and pre-eclampsia can make a woman prone to heart disease, diabetes or high blood pressure for the rest of her life but they aren't always kept under close watch. What is more heavily scrutinised is snapping back into shape or the change in the external appearance of the new body.

Losing baby weight is popular with so-called weight-loss experts. Former Australian *The Biggest Loser* trainer Michelle Bridges has a program called *12WBT* (12-week body transformation), on her website, which includes a post-partum section advising new mums not to diet and then proceeds to list diet advice such as ditching all junk food and keeping a food diary. (Because new mothers have so much time to analyse every morsel of food they eat!) She also advises breastfeeding for weight loss – a common and popular weight-loss method suggested by everyone from family and friends to bloggers alike. Breastfeeding is most importantly a healthy and cheap way to feed your baby and has a whole host of benefits for everyone. By all means though, let's make sure we focus on how breastfeeding can help you 'snap back into shape' quickly, as if there isn't enough pressure around breastfeeding already. This kind of advice deprioritises the health benefits for mother and baby and adds yet another layer of guilt to those who find they can't breastfeed.

A belly wrap or a kind of post-partum garter belt is also popularised by some 'experts' (I am disgusted at myself for even referring to them as such). There is no evidence that these belts improve weight loss; in fact, they can be uncomfortable and place unnecessary pressure on internal organs. They may help mothers who have had a caesarean and are experiencing pain, but mummy tummies are a combination of a big uterus, weight and fluid gain, and abdominal muscle changes. You can do sit-ups all day long and wear a waist trainer all you like, but some of those changes don't go away easily.

Even before baby arrives, super-fit mums-to-be share posts of putting their body through its paces. A number of popular mothers-to-be show videos of their modified workouts, where they exercise with a neat little baby bump in a two-piece outfit. Fitness model Sarah Stage made headlines around the world when, at nine months pregnant, she shared a photo of herself in lingerie, still with abs. A study of magazines for pregnant women found that a substantial proportion of advertisements for pregnant women were about post-partum weight-loss diets and even sexualised the woman's body. A number of these pictures aren't even of women who have had children – they're models! These body types are most definitely not typical for what most expectant mothers see, with typical weight gain for pregnancy between 7–11.5 kilograms.

Working out in pregnancy is also a damned-if-you-do, damned-if-you-don't situation, with mothers who are pregnant and exercising sometimes subject to public criticism for exercising and endangering the baby. Australian personal trainer and CrossFit coach Revie Jane Schulz continued exercising at a safe level during her pregnancy; her posts of her workouts were littered with comments as to how irresponsible she was being with her unborn child's life. Similarly, Kayla Itsines was faced with trolling over her decision to keep working out (safely, mind you) during pregnancy.

There is a lot of misinformation about what is and isn't healthy, and even what is normal or achievable, when it comes to what you do and what you look like when babies are in the mix. Exercise and healthy eating should absolutely be encouraged in pregnant women, new mothers and not-so-new mothers. The list of benefits of exercise in pregnancy is not small and includes maintaining fitness, agility and strength and avoiding excessive weight gain in pregnancy, which is associated with gestational diabetes and larger babies. Big babies put mum and baby at risk for complications during delivery. Exercise also helps with the aches and pains of pregnancy and reduces the risk of serious pregnancy illness such as diabetes and preeclampsia. Exercise obviously needs to be safe for women too and they need to avoid falls, jumping, exercising in high heat and getting the heart rate too high. We see similar benefits for keeping nutritionally sound in pregnancy and, despite being told that we're eating for two, new mums only need to increase their calorie intake by around 340–450 additional calories a day as well as keeping an eye on important micronutrients such as iron, calcium, vitamin D and folic acid.

Here's a really important thing though. Not exercising enough in pregnancy is not a failure of mum to care enough about herself or her baby. In fact, a review of over 20 years of research into exercise in pregnancy showed that the most reliable predictors of a woman exercising during pregnancy were related to higher education, income, no other kids to look after, being white and previously being active. That is: privilege. So why are we constantly hammering women who don't exercise for not caring enough about themselves? We should be helping them to be healthy, not shaming them into doing it. It also means that the constant pressure from the media or Instagram to stay or snap back into shape are superficial; like most aspects of diet culture, this is the realm of a perceived massive personal moral failure rather than something linked to your circumstances and your biology, both of which can be hard to fight. Wanting to wear a bikini after having a baby is not enough to overcome either of these things, despite what fitness 'experts' tell you.

The US National Academy of Medicine states that after pregnancy, about half of women retain more than 5.4 kg and a quarter over 9.1 kg. Nobody is quite sure how quickly the weight can be lost but some experts suggest it will take at least 6–12 months to lose weight at a rate of 0.5 kg per week at most. Breastfeeding does show some small advantage in losing weight but doesn't fully replace the importance of a healthful diet and exercise. Exercise in particular may help lessen any depressive symptoms after pregnancy. And just as with anyone who has not given birth, steering clear of diets may well be important in reducing disordered eating and binge eating. One study published in the *Maternal and Child Health Journal* actually found that intuitive eating was beneficial for new mothers with more loss of the pregnancy weight which has the distinct advantage of avoiding disordered eating and being a lot less arduous than dieting for new mothers.

It's absolutely vital that everyone gets moving, eats well, manages stress and all of the other things we need to do to be healthy. However, the constant pressure on pregnant women and mums to do so really focuses on getting back a pre-baby body, rather than their health. Aided by celebrity photos and diet and exercise plans aimed at new mums, the pressure is harmful. These expectations are usually unrealistic, like most 'body fixes', and ignore the permanency of some changes that happen after giving birth.

Trying to say that you can 'get your body back' shows a lack of understanding and a lack of sympathy for those who have bigger changes after the baby and ignores the fact that a woman's body will rarely be exactly the same after pregnancy. The expectations are not focused on function and what the body can achieve, since that body just grew, housed and birthed a whole human; it seems wrong to turn it around and make it all about looks. All of a sudden, we go from the beauty and miracle of having children to a notion that the body is ruined and that, short of an immense commitment, women are letting themselves go in the wake of having kids. None of this actually helps mums to be healthy. In fact, it leads to poor mental and physical health, disordered eating and less exercise. And, of course, that intense body dissatisfaction is at risk of being passed along to the kids and then the cycle starts all over again.

Pregnant women and mothers need our support to be healthy, not to be yummy mummies. They need to be able to be healthy and help baby be healthy, rather than being concerned with losing the baby weight, snapping back into shape or breastfeeding the pounds away. Pregnancy and motherhood is the ultimate example of where the pressure to look good is disguised as advice to be healthy. In fact, in some instances, the 'advice' given to mums is barely masquerading as health advice. The crappy and harmful information given at what is often a vulnerable time has got to stop being about looks. Instead it needs to be about health and the future of the mother and child – and this means it should stay out of the hands of people who aren't actually there to help with health.

When your health really is at stake

For those of us who have been fortunate enough to have generally pretty good health, being healthy is probably just like it says in the magazine; it's being slim, active, looking alert and feeling energetic. If you aren't #blessed, as social media tends to say at every opportunity, then health can look a little different for you. Given that I am surrounded by people who are sometimes incredibly sick, I started to wonder whether having an illness changes your perceptions on life. I once heard athlete and motivational speaker Turia Pitt talk about the life-threatening burn injury she suffered during an ultra-marathon. She joked that she was 'looking damn fine' before and that she thinks she looks 'damn fine' after. Then again, she was told she may not walk again and now she does Ironman triathlons, so I think she embodies the kind of love and appreciation for her body that a lot of us wish we had.

People who have experienced a major illness or injury are faced with changes in their bodies, which can take them far away from the thin, beautiful ideal. Suddenly, their body is not their own and is poked, cut and injected in an effort to sometimes save their life. Medical teaching tells us that we value, in this order, life then limb then function and finally form. Not everyone sees it this way and nor should they. Just like in breast cancer, it's vital not to trivialise appearance concerns. However, for people who have had injuries or illness that have resulted in them, for example, having a spinal cord injury or an amputation, function is vitally important. Then the focus on their body's abilities can be significant and also lead to a sense of independence and accomplishment. For me, this just hammers home how resilient our sense of our ability is, even in much more challenging situations than many of us will face.

I spend much of my days with people whose bodies have changed irrevocably from illness. Many of them are scarred, some are swollen and others have very visible differences. I've seen this in young people who have a stoma, which we do to divert the bowel to the skin; their fecal matter is collected in a bag they wear on their abdomen. I've seen weight gain and bloated faces in transplant recipients who take life-saving medications to stop their organ being rejected. I always notice that they are not blind to their changing bodies but everyone's reaction is slightly different. Some fight against image standards – wearing a bikini even with a stoma bag in an attempt to normalise it – and others just see it as part and parcel of their illness and recovery. Either way, health has shifted from being solely about being beautiful and therefore healthy to actually being healthy. Very few people know the true value of health the way someone who has a serious illness does.

Research has shown that some people who have had cancer or a transplant, for example, use this as a defining moment in their life. Some studies of those who have survived cancer report that these people have increased vitality, redefined priorities and positive behavioural changes. They know what health means and they are holding on to it like never before. This can have important benefits for their physical health. This was shown in a study of women with breast cancer who were taught stress reduction: they had lowered levels of the stress hormone cortisol, which could help them resist the way stress challenges their physical health, particularly their immune system. In people who have received a kidney transplant, a major surgery and lifelong commitment to medications and check-ups, there is a phenomenon called benefit finding where people identify positive psychological benefits after something negative or traumatic. One of the ways in which they benefit from this serious illness is to have an awareness of their own physical and emotional health.

It makes complete sense. People who have had a serious illness frequently say that they are so appreciative of their health, of being cancer free, or off dialysis if they have received a kidney transplant.

My heart-transplant patients, some of whom wait for a transplant while on a mechanical heart, are thrilled to go swimming, something they haven't been able to do with their lifesaving machine. It's about their health and ability and, while appearance does matter and factor into their wellbeing, I find this phenomenon a reminder that there is so much in the world that is more important than fitting the beautiful ideal. That isn't health: this is.

Placing importance on appearance does not make you a superficial or a bad person but 'beauty' is tenuous and it can be fleeting. It also does not equate to health in the same way that the experience of someone who has has cancer or has been in an accident knows health. Health to them is much more than that. If there was any way to unhook the notion that health equals beauty, this would have to be it.

Chapter 9

PRETTY HEALTHY

'Don't let some motivational quote make you feel bad about yourself.'

DR NIKKI STAMP

Although our society appears to be obsessed with health, that's really not the case. As we've found out, the reasons are complex, but most of us aren't doing what we need to. The result is that we're pretty unhealthy.

I remember sitting at the gate at Heathrow Airport when this idea hit me: one of the reasons health is still such a struggle for so many of us is that we're busy trying to be pretty instead of healthy. From having a single thought about why we're still struggling with preventable diseases and why I try to help people with that every day, I went down a pathway that confirmed my worst fears: that our idea of health and the way in which it's promoted is broken. I had no idea of the extent to which we're almost universally failed by the health messages we receive, from governments and health professionals right down to the ones we flick past on Instagram.

Our health and wellbeing are the most important things any of us will ever have and it's time to take back control of our physical and mental condition from the wrong people. It's far too important to keep going in the same direction; one that has made it hard for us to differentiate between real and fake information, between real health and just looking a certain way.

You are too important to be left up to a social media influencer, a sportswear brand or a weight-loss program.

In my job, I have to earn people's trust. I know that it may not seem that way, given doctors are still deferred to, but I have to look people in the eye and tell them why my treatment is going to help them. I have to explain why they should trust me to make them better, take away their pain or save their life and they, in turn, have to agree to that. There isn't a brand or influencer on the planet who has to do that: earn trust in that way. But our health is being treated by many people who seek and get our blind trust on flimsy promises and bad science. Every time someone tries to do that in future, I want you to remember that you are too valuable and your health is too precious to give it up for quick fixes, false hopes and being pretty. And with that in mind, I want us all to take back our health from the many people who don't value it as we do.

Big Wellness

Going through hundreds of social media posts, blogs, podcasts and documentaries to discover what ridiculous health information is out in the world has made me angry. Every time I see some charlatan saying you can 'cure cancer' or 'detoxify your liver' or 'get your best body yet' through some ludicrous diet or exercise program, I feel my blood pressure rise. Every time I see a post on how you can transform yourself in time for your summer bikini body, I am disappointed for the thousands of women, men and children who see this and are made to feel bad about themselves. Every time I see some quasi-scientific statement that has absolutely no truth in the matter, I feel angry and then almost powerless to fight against the growing tide of crap that pretends to want to make us healthy but is doing the exact opposite.

It feels feeble to try to fight back against the noise of bad health advice that is now predominantly available online. There is a complete lack of accountability over what information is being put out there and what it does to people. If doctors or other health professionals made frivolous claims about medicine and surgery, like the diet, exercise and wellness gurus do, we would be vilified. Actually, we would be disciplined. And quite correctly, because we have no right to play with people's health and wellbeing. We have no right to play off people's hope or fears to advance our own ego or simply to get paid. When a doctor pushes a treatment in the same way people do online, there are vocal critics who slam us for 'being in bed with Big Pharma' or pushing our own agenda at the expense of the patient.

Big Wellness is absolutely no different. Make no mistake, just like any other multi-billion-dollar industry, it wants to continue to make billions of dollars, grow its business and satisfy shareholders. Individuals still want fame and fortune. That's not to say that some of these people don't have genuinely good intentions but their ignorance of the damage they could be doing or that there could be a better way to help others is no longer enough of an excuse. Whenever you look at someone selling a diet, or a supplement or an exercise program, they might actually want to help you. But you can bet a number of them are in it for the cash and don't give a damn about you once they have your admiration, 'likes' and money. Don't think that because they're not obviously attached to some big company, or that they feel weirdly connected to you, that they care for you. They don't. Big Wellness has too much skin in the game to actually care about how much healthier and better off you are.

The inaccurate and sometimes harmful information that we're sold about our health is perfect in the age of social media. Social media and the internet have created an unprecedented ability to exert influence over a wider audience than ever before. And, sadly, that influence often carries information that can be anything from wrong to damaging to downright dangerous. People can genuinely be harmed by misinformation or by placing trust in the wrong people or wrong ideals.

It wasn't Belle Gibson's false health claims that brought her undone, because it seemed wrong to question a young woman apparently fighting for her life. What brought her lies crashing down was the fact that she had not paid large sums to charity despite claiming she was fundraising for them. With regards to her health claims, the possibility that people may have shunned life-saving yet dreadfully un-Instagrammable and proven medical treatment was a side dish to her fraud.

Just wanting it more?

Not only is health – especially looking healthy – the latest trend that we covet, it's given rise to a kind of moral superiority around being healthy. You get what you work for, you get the body you deserve. So, someone with cancer deserves it? Someone who had a heart attack, well, they had it coming? The appearance of health is so strongly desired that if you live a perfect, healthy, smoothie-fuelled life, you are deemed to be far morally superior to the person who falls short of this standard.

To be healthy, what we really need is a combination of good genetics, a nutritious diet, exercise and psychological wellbeing. It's as simple and as difficult as that. Even though the pathway to health seems to be made up of these relatively straightforward building blocks, they do not happen in isolation. Our ability or our interest to engage in these healthy behaviours is not simply a matter of wanting it more. One of the biggest predictors of health is our environment; health does not happen in a vacuum. Not everyone is afforded the same privilege of being able to use the latest Instagram trainer's workout or buy the new expensive superfood. Some people struggle to exercise because they have nowhere safe to do so or they're working multiple jobs just to put food, any food, on the table.

In Australia, the 20 per cent of people who live in the lowest socioeconomic area are 1.6 times as likely to have a chronic illness as the 20 per cent living in the most affluent areas. People without privilege have smaller babies, are more likely to put off seeing a doctor for economic reasons, spend less on health and medical care, and even die earlier. And yet to improve your health all you need to do is want it more, according to some people.

If only the individuals and big businesses who carry on about wanting to make people healthier through their revolutionary training process or extraordinary diet would make it available to everyone who needs it. This would show some insight into the fact that determination is not the only thing that it takes; a whole host of other factors need to fall into place. Our governments and workplaces and community would get together and make sure that everybody, no matter where they lived, could access the seemingly simple things we all need to be healthy. We would eradicate the biases that make it hard to be healthy.

But they don't. The inequalities that contribute to ill health are everywhere and a shiny Instagram post telling you to love yourself enough to exercise is not going to change all of that.

For those who share real, good-quality scientific information, the landscape has changed irrevocably. Now scientists and health-care professionals are not only trying to get the right information out there, they have to defend it from an onslaught of inaccurate advice because the pendulum has swung away from science and medicine. A 2016 US Gallup report indicates that only 36 per cent of Americans have trust in the medical system. Why don't we apply that same scepticism to wellness bloggers? Why is Gwyneth Paltrow's *Goop* growing at a mind-blowing rate, selling vaginal steamers? (Incidentally, the vagina is a self-cleaning organ and doesn't need boiling–hot water blown at it for health or beauty.) For years, science and medicine have had to prove themselves but there is such a distrust of medicine and its slow progress and lack of quick fixes that we're in an era when we'd rather risk third-degree burns to our genitals than listen to actual qualified experts, because their advice is old news or downright boring.

Science is not a collection of immutable facts; it is a persistent advancement of our knowledge. Nutrition science is constantly evolving as are psychology, medicine and exercise science. Every day, I know I can learn something new about the human body, something that we didn't know before. Sometimes that new knowledge will make something else seem completely wrong. Science has been wrong in the past and it will be wrong again. That doesn't mean it's to be distrusted. Science naturally evolves and updates, which means things change. That is absolutely okay, even if at times it's confusing. Now we live in a world where some influencers' opinions are more important than well-conducted research. This is anti-intellectualism coupled with capitalism and it's putting our wellbeing at risk.

While it's hard to police, there have to be some standards set for what is being said. I once tried to report an Instagram account that was sharing utter garbage about the way liver disease could be cured with a vegetable juice, among other medically inaccurate information. However, I couldn't report it because it wasn't impersonating a person, it wasn't spam and it wasn't annoying. I couldn't even report an anti-vaxxer account for spreading harmful information, which it is. How is this even possible? You can post something on social media, have it seen by countless people, shared and go viral and there is absolutely no recourse or reporting mechanism available to stop it from causing harm. By the time someone has been able to write a rebuttal, it's too late because that original post has been seen and shared more times than can be rebutted.

To attack social media as the root of all of our health problems would be a gross oversimplification. Social media is just the latest way to share information; it presents new and unique challenges, but at its essence it's just the same shit, different day. Diets and exercise programs or notions of beauty have been spread around for years by the media, by our families and by our friendship groups. Publishing on social media is rapid and very reliant on imagery that amplifies its impact. It is also less regulated than mainstream media, so the quality of information can be even worse. We are still learning to harness its power for good; when it comes to our health, we need to get on and maximise the benefits and minimise the harm.

As much as I would like to see swindlers of the world vanish into thin air, I have to be sensible. Social media and the people and corporations who have built a business around telling us that we're not healthy/pretty enough aren't going anywhere. Models are not all of the sudden going to disappear or at least start looking like the average human. Photoshop is not going to vanish – if anything, the constant stream of apps on your phone to make you look better will keep coming. Companies will still pay influencers to sell quick fixes like teas to flatten your tummy. Human nature dictates that we will still look wistfully at pictures of slender models and want to be like that. I do, however, believe that there is a better message to give to people to put a stop to our reliance on non-experts and our obsession with beauty and all that this entails. I believe that we can be healthier and we can unhook the claws of Big Wellness from our backs and do better than what we're currently doing.

Despite what popular bloggers, social media stars and trainers would have you believe, health is not about making you more beautiful. Is there anything wrong with wanting to look better? No. But let's stop pretending we're selling health when we talk about glowing skin, white teeth, tiny waists and bikini bodies. That is not health. Selling good nutrition or exercise as a judgement on beauty or morality is making us unhealthier, not healthier; so stop bullshitting the population and be real with what you're actually telling people. Be real with what you're telling yourself.

The bulk of evidence shows us that, despite best intentions, being motivated by image is probably harmful to our mental and physical health. It doesn't sustain motivation and it's probably as damaging to self-worth as watching a catwalk model. So why the hell do we buy into it?

Because beauty is not just a commodity to want, it is *the* commodity to want. Our society has evolved to make sure that beauty is valued above all else and, because of that, your attractiveness has become associated with everything from what sort of a person you are to your worth in life. It's a tool used to keep people down and now we use that to make judgements, including moral ones on how healthy someone else is, how healthy we are. If our body isn't beautiful in a bikini, we're not worthy of being seen, we're not worthy of good things and we're not as healthy as we should be. We're bad people.

Get curious: how to spot an actual expert

Given the fact that any Sally Selfie can tell you what to do online for your body, one of the first steps in conquering the unhealthy messages out there is to learn how to sort the real from the fake. I like to think of this as curiosity. When you click on something or pick up a magazine, access that curiosity to go beyond what is presented to you as gospel truth. Some days and with some messages, that curiosity is more like straight-out scepticism.

The first question to ask is, who is telling you this bit of information? My favourite example is still the American man who gets his social media 'health information' delivered to him by a spirit. Just to clarify, information that appears to have been obtained from a ghost is bad. From a truly qualified expert, it can be great. You need to know if that person is actually qualified to talk about and advise you on that topic. Qualifications don't come based on numbers of followers or book sales, and they don't universally extend outside the boundaries of their area of expertise, such as personal trainers giving out nutrition information or nutritionists prescribing exercise programs. It's great that people have opinions, but their experience researched by Googling some blogs and doing a six-week detox does not better the information from people who actually know what they're talking about.

A big red flag for me is whether or not their advice or opinions are in line with accepted thinking. For example, if someone is advocating cutting out whole groups of foods or claiming to cure cancer in a way that is opposed by mainstream experts, we need to be wary of what they're saying. Don't get me wrong: science and accepted thinking needs to be challenged for it to evolve and for us to learn more. But if it's way out of left field, something could be wrong. Miracle cures, guarantees and sure-fire anything fall into this category. There is very little in this world that is guaranteed, so when someone says 'sure-fire', call bullshit on that. That includes some of the science around nutrition, exercise, weight loss and health in general. There are still many shades of grey and unanswered questions about what we do; being able to admit that is evidence of someone who *does* understand what they do.

We often place a lot of faith in individual experience but anecdotes are not scientific data. Just because Instagram Imogen did a juice cleanse that made her skin glow or Betty Burpee has sculpted the juiciest booty yet with her workout does not mean it will work for you. Quite the opposite in fact; people have varied needs and wants when it comes to their health and what works for one person won't always work for someone else. Claiming it did work doesn't mean much when it comes to saying that a health product is worthwhile. Backing up a claim requires high-quality, rigorous scientific research. One Instagram post does not equal science.

Having the science to back it up is vital when it comes to making choices for your health. If you ask someone to support the claims they're making and they argue with you, avoid backing it up, cite individual experiences or make you feel bad for daring to question their internet-given authority, then beware. People who are delivering you real honest-to-goodness, scientific solutions can back up what they're saying with information that has come from the highest levels of scientific investigation; they'll do so happily and admit where there are gaps in their knowledge.

And, of course, if it seems too good to be true, it probably is.

Look for reputable information from websites and social media accounts run by people and organisations that genuinely have some expertise. Keep in mind that it can be hard to work out what is real and what's not, so if you're not sure, reach out to an expert: your doctor, nutritionist, dietitian, or a qualified trainer, amongst many others.

Unravelling the confusing world of media

Evaluating the media has got to be one of the most important skills we need in this modern life of ours. Research suggests that media literacy, an ability to critically evaluate and interpret the messages the media presents to us, is vitally important in protecting us against confusing or damaging information. This isn't just about shutting out inaccurate messages, it's about protecting ourselves from the unwanted side effects of seeing bikini bodies and diet culture everywhere.

This is an important skill because, although we might like policing of media and social media, it's probably not going to happen; either because it's too damn hard to do or because it's not in the commercial interests of the media organisations. It's not excusable, because I think we all know that the media and social media can do better. But media literacy can provide a buffer against the harm caused by some images.

This truncated method of evaluating media comes from the National Eating Disorder Association and, while it's obviously geared towards body image, disordered eating and eating disorders, the broad principles stay the same. When you look at a magazine article, TV ad or social media post, start by asking who made the article or the post. Look at their motivations behind it: are they selling something, entertaining you or providing information? Look at any techniques used to make the message such as photoshopping, celebrity endorsement or models posing as real people – are these real-life or unattainable? And, of course, how does this make you feel? If you feel guilty, bad about yourself, inadequate or inferior, even if the message is well intended, it's not for you so give it a miss.

Cultivating an awareness about what media in any form would have us believe is a skill and once you start looking, not only will you get better at it, you will be shocked at how much of what you see online, on TV or in magazines doesn't pass the test. It doesn't mean that you will be left with nothing to scroll through at night or no magazines to read; it just means that you look at what you're shown with a discerning eye, empowering you to take what you need for your wellbeing and leave behind what you don't.

Putting it all together: how to be pretty healthy

❶ UNFOLLOW AND DISENGAGE

In order to write this book, I had to go behind enemy lines in a sense. I followed many social media accounts that advertised flat-tummy teas, weight-loss lollipops and posted daily pictures of someone working out in a crop top. Bonus points if the captions included some motivational quote like 'Summer bodies are made in the winter' or 'Don't wish for a good body, work for it'. (Those quotes made me wish to throw up in my mouth a little bit.) I promised myself that by the time I finished writing I would unfollow all of them, but I didn't last that long. I became so sick of the lies and the fact that I felt bad about myself or unmotivated that I cut them out of my life early. And that was the absolute best piece of research I did for this book.

Since the message that we're not enough is fairly common and sometimes hard to avoid, I think it's important to take back control where we can. Just knowing that diet advertising is bad for us doesn't mean it will go away. It will always remain hard to avoid billboards or other ads but we can control what we choose to pay attention to. Think of it not only as a spring clean for your Instagram but a new chance for your mind and body. While scrolling through or just being online, notice what makes you feel good about yourself and what makes you feel bad. And if it makes you feel a little bad, then disengage. Same goes for anything else that gives you that 'I'm not as pretty/slim/healthy/fit/strong as they are' and comes with that uncomfortable feeling of shame. Get rid of it.

Instead of following dozens of fitness goddesses or dieting accounts, why not branch out? Start following people who love their bodies, because it's infectious. Look at men, women and transgender people of different racial backgrounds, of different sizes and of different abilities to see all the glorious ways human bodies can be. Check out people who can do amazing things and inspire you do the same. Follow scientists and health experts who will give you a much better idea of what you can aim for rather than slim, rich, white women who got rich off your insecurities and are slim because of their genetics and then photoshopped to perfection. Stay on social media, but fill your feed with people who make you smarter, happier, healthier and feel good about yourself.

❷ EAT FOR YOUR HEALTH AND ENJOYMENT

Food has become a loaded topic. Foods are good or bad, healthy or unhealthy. They're reduced to protein or antioxidants or calories or, even worse, medicine. The connotations and expectations that surround food have taken away what I think are its two true values:

we need the energy from food to make our bodies work; and food should be enjoyable. We use to it to celebrate, to commiserate, to convey culture, or just simply because it tastes good.

A little along the lines of the intuitive eating principle of 'gentle nutrition', eating for your health also has to encompass eating for enjoyment. Where possible, eat good, healthful foods like vegetables, fruits, whole grains and proteins to fuel your body. Keep in mind though that food does not have to look picture perfect to be healthy. Nor do you have to eat clean all the time. Food should bring you nourishment as well as enjoyment or social connection. So don't buy into the shame of eating carbs or cake or whatever it is that you want. A good diet is about what you do *most* of the time and you are much more likely to eat well when you stop depriving yourself of certain foods.

❸ MOVE YOUR BODY TO BE STRONG

Exercise is great for the mind, body and soul. It protects your physical health, your mental health and can allow you to stay engaged with other people, all of which are important for health and sustaining interest. Instead of exercising to punish yourself, exercise and feel how remarkable your body is. How it can run or walk, swim or dance. Focus on what your body is doing, not what it looks like.

❹ DO WHAT BRINGS YOU SATISFACTION AND ENJOYMENT

There is overwhelming evidence that when you embark on a change for your health, you are more likely to stick it out if you steer clear of external motivators. Don't believe it when people tell you all you need is grit or to want it enough. Being motivated for image, or doing something you detest or that you feel you have to do, is not the most likely way to stick at your exercise program.

We need to encourage people to tap into those internal motivators, to find reasons deep down inside for their health. So, don't punish yourself with the exercise you hate most to look good. Find things that satisfy your psyche and bring you enjoyment; they are far more likely to keep you motivated. What does that look like for you? Hunt it down and go for it.

❺ SHOW SOME COMPASSION

Compassion needs to go in two directions. The first is outwards to other people. Bias is so strong in our society and it is impacting on others' ability to be healthy. No matter what we look like, we've probably experienced pressure from other people, whether that be well-meaning advice or something more sinister. Added to this, the further you are from society's ideals of what you should look like, the higher the pressure. That pressure does not do anyone any favours and the impact of bias on the physical and emotional wellbeing of someone subjected to it is inarguable. We have a responsibility to push back and demand that these biases are eradicated, especially in healthcare. The way to do this is to start showing all kinds of ideals, not just a thin, white one. Check your biases and be compassionate towards people who society loves to keep down.

The second way we need to use compassion is inwards, towards ourselves. Self-compassion is emerging as an important psychological buffer that promotes resilience but also helps us actually engage in health-protective behaviour, physical and psychological. Self-compassion is that kind, compassionate and accepting attitude towards yourself during difficult times and is the exact opposite of the 'get your arse off the couch', toughen-up approach that health fanatics would have you believe is the way to change your life. It is not a helpful way to speak to other people and it's certainly not the way to speak to yourself. Compassion isn't about letting yourself off the hook. It's about being kind, acknowledging your shortcomings or even failure in a way that isn't overly emotional and lets you dust yourself off and pick yourself up. Talk to yourself the way you would talk to a friend or a stranger in the street asking for help and tap into your compassion.

⑥ DEMAND A BETTER WORLD

Our health does not happen in a vacuum. You can do all the burpees, eat all the vegetables and practise self-compassion all damn day but it does not change the world around us. The world around us is broken when it comes to our health. There are far too many things working directly against our health and wellbeing; to make a truly healthy world, those things have to change.

The fashion industries and mass media markets have listened to what the people wanted, even if it's only a little bit. There have been changes in standards of models used, inclusion of diverse body shapes and sizes, better representation of people of colour and less use and greater acknowledgment of photo editing. They're pretty small changes that don't yet make a big enough dent, but they do, however, illustrate something important: we have the power to demand more from people, organisations and governments. We have the power to demand whatever it is that needs to change for us to be healthy.

While getting fashion industries to change is a coup, there is much more left to do, so many more people to be held accountable. If I had my way, people would *never* be allowed to advertise dietary supplements on social media, especially when those people are celebrities or being paid the big bucks to say something will 'fix' your body. Social media and mainstream media would responsibly police what's posted online and if someone were lying in a way that impacts people's health, those posts or news items would be disallowed. Advertising would be transparent and inclusive. Governments would institute preventative health programs that took into account the huge and impactful social determinants of health, which cannot be overcome by a TV ad telling you to eat more vegetables if all you can afford is the fast food down the road.

These are lofty goals and I know they may not be reached any time soon. However, we cannot underestimate the power of a groundswell. What might start as one little voice, questioning the messages given, rebelling against diet culture and not starving herself, or asking friends not to engage in fat talk, can grow. Imagine if friends and family started to follow suit, then her workplace, which then escalated to include the community, the country and so on.

We can all start being that change by disengaging from those behaviours that perpetuate diet culture, prioritise appearance and devalue actual health. Tell your friends that you're going to stop giving compliments on weight loss or appearance. We have to start small with this because taking back our health is a big fight.

Even the smallest actions can change the world; today, I hope you take even the smallest step to make yourself and the whole world pretty healthy.

EPILOGUE

✦ ✦ ✦

I still have moments when I recall the advice that personal trainer gave me about food. That potatoes are bad and that only certain fruits were compatible with looking a particular way. I like sweet potatoes, but I would always look sideways at a potato with the mantra in my head 'potatoes are bad, potatoes are bad' on repeat. It took away from the enjoyment of a really good roast dinner. It meant that one of my favourite fruits, bananas, were consumed with a good slice of guilt. Not anymore. I love potatoes, I like roasting them, mashing them, I bloody well like eating them and now I do. Same with bananas and pineapple, which had once been banished to the 'bad' side of the equation. Now I can enjoy nutritious food – actually most food – guilt-free. Fear has been used for too long to sell poor-quality information but now the only thing I'm afraid of is continuing to mess up my mind with lists of 'should's and should not's'.

I had a beautiful big bowl of pasta last night and that would normally mean I would have to go running to work off the carbs. I did go running this morning. I laced up my shoes and started my shuffle around a picturesque park, complete with ducks and sunrise made of a beautiful pallet of golds, pinks and purples. I enjoyed the air on my face, the sounds of the wildlife and the smell of the native Australian trees. I enjoyed the entire experience and for me it meant I began my day with a smile on my face. I ran for enjoyment, for the sensory enjoyment of everything

I experienced. I ran for my health and for a sense of accomplishment and achievement. And I also ran because I wanted to feel like I looked good and to fit into clothes and to beat my last time on this particular route. All the research and delving into why we want to be healthy has not completely erased decades of conditioning that beauty is health and to be pursued at all costs. Honestly though, when my alarm went off, I wanted to roll over and ignore it and spend just a few more minutes in the warmth and comfort of my bed. But I still went.

Writing this book has been a deep dive for me into the world of health, body image, what we do poorly and what we do well. At times, it has been a confronting look at my own life, including my own motivations for taking care of myself or how I can be so demanding on myself, constantly insisting on perfection. It's also been somewhat uncomfortable to learn what we in the health-care system do poorly and what we can do better. I've followed social media accounts that have felt like poison just to see what the general public is being told. And of course, examining all of these things in the context of a world that isn't necessarily set up to help us be healthy has at times been frustrating. It has been hard not to be infuriated with the people, the companies and even the government forces that do not promote or prioritise our health and instead distribute misinformation, place profit above people or simply fail to do the right thing.

It's easy to spiral down into this frustration and let it take over, but this has never really been my approach to life. I have always felt that by exposing the problems at hand and looking at the science and the evidence, then we have half a chance of prevailing. And that is exactly how I feel at the end of this book. Writing it has given me so much new information and I am grateful for the opportunity to share that on these pages, and with the people around me. I have also changed things about the way I talk to people when I see them in my hospital and I hope I have done them right in helping them on the path to be healthy. I know not everyone will agree with me. I know that this may well be debated and disagreed with. But I hope that this book sparks conversations and curiosity around all of the things that we're doing that are harming us, not helping.

On a personal note, I am every person who has felt negative about their body. How it looks or how it works. I have faced my own health and illness while at the same time looking at them through the lens of beauty or fatness and thinness. I have fought in my own head a battle between knowing the science and being swayed by the seductiveness of beauty and health messages. Writing this book has made me face up to my own beliefs, my own demons and my own pursuit of health. It has made me look critically at the system I work in and yearn for a time when we can do better to support people's health holistically, not just fighting disease but creating health in all its forms.

Most of all, since writing this book, I have learnt to be kinder to myself, even if only just a little. And that kindness has translated into better physical and mental wellbeing. I have unfollowed vast numbers of Instagram accounts when I realised that they sold promises of magic bullets and pseudoscience and that looking at them created a pit in my stomach – they made me think I was not good enough. I now look at food as nutrition and something to be enjoyed, rather than something that is good or bad. I stopped punishing my mind and body and started looking at all the science and research that I had discovered that showed me a better, healthier way of living. In my mind things feel that little bit clearer. I feel empowered to embrace the complexities of my thoughts and to pursue a wholly happy and healthy life. It is my most sincere and deepest hope that you do too.

SUGGESTED READINGS
AND REFERENCES

✦ ✦ ✦

Below is a list of resources that I have found to be enlightening, useful or a challenge to the way we think about health, diet culture, exercise and body image.

BOOKS

Embrace Yourself
Taryn Brumfitt (also check out
Embrace: The Documentary)

Just Eat It
Laura Thomas PhD

Run Like A Girl
Alexandra Heminsley

Big Fit Girl
Louise Green

Body Positive Power
Megan Jayne Crabbe

The Beauty Myth
Naomi Wolf

Hunger
Roxane Gay

The Woman Who Fooled The World
Beau Donelly and Nick Toscano

*The Mindful Self-Compassion
Workbook: A Proven Way
to Accept Yourself and Build Inner
Strength and Thrive*
Kristin Neff and Christopher Germer

Bad Science
Ben Goldacre

Rising Strong
Brené Brown

WEBSITES

Body Confident Mums (*I cannot
recommend this website and program
enough*)
https://www.bodyconfidentmums.org

Mayo Clinic
http://www.mayoclinic.com

Heart Foundation (Australia)
https://www.heartfoundation.org.au/

British Heart Foundation
https://www.bhf.org.uk/

Centre for Appearance Research
https://www1.uwe.ac.uk/hls/
research/appearanceresearch.aspx

Self Determination Theory
http://selfdeterminationtheory.org

The Butterfly Foundation
https://thebutterflyfoundation.org.au

NCDFree
http://ncdfree.org

Lyndi Cohen: *The Nude Nutritionist*
https://www.lyndicohen.com

The Rooted Project
https://www.therootedproject.co.uk

Dr Zali Yager (*Body image and eating disorder prevention researcher*)
https://www.zaliyager.com

PODCASTS

Science Vs
Hosted by Wendy Zuckerman, Science Vs breaks down the science behind many modern myths, with health-related topics featuring regularly. It's funny and informative.

All In The Mind
Hosted by Lyn Malcolm, this podcast explores important psychology and brain-related science and is fascinating and informative listening.

Nutrition Matters – Paige Smathers – Registered Dietitian
Smathers investigates the ins and outs of food and nutrition from a diet-free framework.

Appearance Matters: The Podcast – The Centre for Appearance Research
From UK body image researchers, this podcast really delves deep into body image and how it affects our health and wellbeing.

SOCIAL MEDIA ACCOUNTS

Body Image Movement (Taryn Brumfitt)
@bodyimage movement

The Nude Nutritionist
@nude_nutritionist

The Rooted Project
@therootedproject

Alan Flanagan, Nutritional Advocate
@thenutritional_advocate

Dr Katherine Iscoe
@dr_katherine

Lucy Mountain
@thefashionfitnessfoodie

I Weigh
@i_weigh

Bo Stanley
@bostanley

Megan Jayne Crabbe
@bodyposipanda

Tally
@tallyrye

Danny Lennon
@dannylennon_sigma

Celeste Barber
@celestebarber

Savina Rego, The Savy Dietitian
@thesavydietitian

Revie Jane Schultz
@reviejane

Kimberley Wilson
@foodandpsych

Fight the Fads
@fightthefads

This Girl Can
@thisgirlcanuk

Girls Make Your Move
@girlsmakeyourmove

Ashlee Bennett
@bodyimage_therapist

Laura Thomas PhD
@laurathomasphd

Athletics Not Aesthetics
@athleticsnotaesthetics

What Mia Did Next
@whatmiadidnext

Joanne Encarnacion
@gofitjo

Positively Glittered
@positivelyglittered

Dr Megan Rossi RD APD
@theguthealthdoctor

Body Positive Fitness
@bodypositivefitness_

Eva, What's My Body Doing?
@whatsmybodydoing

Untrap
@untrapped_au

Dr Ciara Kelly
@theirishbalance

Beauty Redefined – Lindsay &
Lexie Kite, PhD
@beauty_redefined

Dr Joshua Wolrich
@drjoshuawolrich

Dr Hazel Wallace, The Food Medic
@thefoodmedic

Grace Woodward
@gracewoodward

Nadia Craddock
@nadia.craddock

Maeve Hanan
@dieteticallyspeaking

Professor Phillippa Diedrichs
@phillippa.diedrichs

Body Confident Mums
@bodyconfidentmums

References by chapter

I've picked a handful of the references, websites and news articles for each chapter that I think constitute important science or vital reading. I have read literally hundreds of journal articles, websites and interviews for this book, containing a wide variety of opinions. The list of references I used is pretty exhaustive, but these ones make for interesting or important reading.

CHAPTER 1: Sick enough yet?

Huber M, Knottnerus et al. (2001) How should we define health?
British Medical Journal

Editorial (2009) What Is Health? *The Lancet*

Australian Institute of Health and Welfare, Australia's Health 2018

Parliament of Australia (2018): Select Committee into the Obesity
Epidemic in Australia.

CHAPTER 2: Why working out isn't working out

2017 State of the UK Fitness Industry Report – Available online –
http://www.leisuredb.com

Nick Mitchell, *The Telegraph*, The diet book industry is a lie – and we've
all been sucked into it. Available online – https://www.telegraph.co.uk

CHAPTER 3: Diet is a four-letter word

Rosie Saunt & Helen West. In Defence of Pre-Made Mash. *Huffington Post.*
Available online – https://www.huffingtonpost.co.uk

The Association of UK Dietitians. *Dietitian, Nutritionist, Nutritional Therapist
or Diet Expert? A comprehensive guide to roles and functions.*

Buchanan K, Sheffield J, Tan WH. (2017) Predictors of diet failure:
A multi-factorial cognitive and behavioral model. *Journal of Health Psychology.*

McEvedy SM, Sullivan-Mort G, McLean SA, Pascoe MC and Paxton SJ. (2017)
Ineffectiveness of commercial weight-loss programs for achieving modest
but meaningful weight loss: Systematic review and meta-analysis.
Journal of Health Psychology.

Hall K. (2013) Diet Versus Exercise in "The Biggest Loser" Weight Loss Competition. *Obesity*.

Fothergill E, Guo J, Howard L et al. (2016) Persistent metabolic adaptation 6 years after 'The Biggest Loser' competition. *Obesity*.

Greenway FL. (2015) Physiological adaptations to weight loss and factors favoring weight gain. *International Journal of Obesity*.

Fardet A, Rock E. (2018) Perspective: Reductionist nutrition research has meaning only within the framework of holistic and ethical thinking. *Advances in Nutrition*.

McKean M, Mitchell L, O'Connor H, Prvan T, Slater G. (2018) Are exercise professionals fit to provide nutrition advice? An evaluation of general nutrition knowledge. *Journal of Science and Medicine in Sport*.

CHAPTER 4: Bikini bodies

Sara Gaynes, Exercise for You, Not Your Looks. *Huffington Post*. Available online – https://www.huffpost.com

Teixeira PJ, Carraca EV, Markland D, Silva MN, Ryan RM. (2012) Exercise, physical activity and self-determination theory: A systematic review. *International Journal of Behavioral Nutrition and Physical Activity*.

Beer NJ, Dimmock JA, Guelfi KJ. (2017) Providing choice in exercise influences food intake at the subsequent meal. *Medicine and Science in Sport and Exercise*.

Raggatt M, Wright CJC, Carotte E, Jenkinson R, Mulgrew K, Prichard I and Lim MSC. (2018) "I aspire to look and feel healthy like the posts convey": engagement with fitness inspiration on social media and perceptions of its influence on health and wellbeing. *BMC Public Health*.

Vartanian LR, Wharton CM, Green EB. (2012) Appearance vs health motives for exercise and for weight loss. *Psychology of Sport and Exercise*.

Burke TJ, Rains SA. (2018) The paradoxical outcomes of observing others' exercise behavior on social network sites: friends' exercise posts, exercise attitudes and weight concern. *Health Communication*.

CHAPTER 5: Eating disorders: the unbearable lightness

Zickgraf HF, Ellis JM, JH Essayli. (2018) Disentangling orthorexia nervosa from healthy eating and other eating disorder symptoms: Relationships with clinical impairment, comorbidity, and self-reported food choices. *Appetite.*

Solmi F, Hatch SL, Hotopf M, Treasure J, Micali N. (2015) Validation of the SCOFF Questionnaire for Eating Disorders in a Multiethnic General Population Sample. *International Journal of Eating Disorders*

Park S (2017) Comparison of body composition between fashion models and women in general. *Journal of Exercise Nutrition and Biochemistry*

Sidani JE, Shensa A, Hoffman B, Hammer J, Primack BA. (2016) The Association between Social Media Use and Eating Concerns among US Young Adults. *Journal of the Academy of Nutrition and Dietetics.*

Mabe A, Fornley KJ, Peel PK. (2014) Do you like my photo? Facebook Use Maintains Eating Disorder Risk. *International Journal of Eating Disorders.*

Holland G, Tiggemann M. (2016). A systematic review of the impact of the use of social networking sites on body image and disordered eating outcomes. *Body Image.*

Colton PA et al. (2015). Eating disorders in girls and women with Type 1 Diabetes: A longitudinal study of prevalence, onset, remission and recurrence. *Diabetes Care.*

Hay P, Chinn D, Forbes D et al. (2014) Royal Australian and New Zealand College of Psychiatrists clinical practice guidelines for the treatment of eating disorders. *Australian and New Zealand Journal of Psychiatry.*

CHAPTER 6: AntiSocial

Berland GK et al. (2001) Health Information on the Internet: Accessibility, quality and reliability in English and Spanish. *JAMA.*

Vogel EA, Rose JP. (2017) Perceptions of Perfection: The influence of social media on interpersonal evaluations. *Basic and Applied Social Psychology.*

Fardouly J, Diedrichs PC, Vartanian LR, Halliwell E. (2015) Social comparisons on social media: The impact of Facebook on young women's body image concerns and mood. *Body Image.*

Tiggemann M, Zaccardo M. (2018) 'Strong is the new skinny': A content analysis of #fitspiration images on Instagram. *Journal of Health Psychology.*

Robinson L, Prichard I, Nikolaidis A, Drummond C, Drummond M, Tiggemann M. (2017) Idealized media images: The effect of fitspiration imagery on body satisfaction and exercise behavior. *Body Image*.

Mulgrew KE, McCulloch K, Farren E, Prichard I, Lim MSC. (2018) This girl can #jointhemovement. Effectiveness of physical functional-focused campaigns for women's body satisfaction and exercise intent. *Body Image*.

'Federal Health Minister Greg Hunt has ordered his department to stop paying social media influencers.' ABC News. Available online: https://www.abc.net.au/news

CHAPTER 7: Body positivity

Sirois FM, Kitner R, Hirsch JK. (2015) Self-compassion, Affect and Health-Promoting Behaviors. *Health Psychology*.

Sainsbury A, Hay P. (2014) Call for an urgent rethink of the 'Health At Every Size' concept. *Journal of Eating Disorders*.

Bacon L, Aphramor L. (2011) Weight Science: Evaluating the Evidence for a Paradigm Shift. *Nutrition Journal*.

Tylka TL, Wood-Baraclow NL. (2015) What is and what is not positive body image? Conceptual foundations and construct definition. *Body Image*.

Brudzynsku L, Ebben WP. (2010) Body Image as a Motivator and Barrier to Exercise Participation. *International Journal of Exercise Science*.

Kelly DeVos – The Problem With Body Positivity. *New York Times*. Available online – https://www.nytimes.com

Pearl RL, Puhl RM. (2018) Weight bias internalization and health: a systematic review. *Obesity Reviews*.

CHAPTER 8: Extraordinary bodies

Leahy K, Berlin K, Banks G, Bachman J. (2017) The Relationship Between Intuitive Eating and Postpartum Weight Loss. *Maternal and Child Health Journal*.

Boepple L, Thompson JK. (2016) An exploration of appearance and health messages present in pregnancy magazines. *Journal of Health Psychology*.

Persson S, Benn Y, Dhingra K, Clark-Carter D, Owen AL, Grogan S. (2018). Appearance-based intervention to reduce UV exposure: A systematic review. *British Journal of Health Psychology.*

McDonnell A, Lin L. (2016) The hot body issue: Weight and caption tone in celebrity gossip magazines. *Body Image.*

Gow RW, Lydecker JA, Lamanna JD, Mazzeo SE. (2012) Representations of celebrities weight and shape during pregnancy and postpartum: A content analysis of three entertainment magazine websites. *Body Image.*

Cousson-Gélie F, Bruchon-Scweitzer M, Dilhuydy JM, Jutand MA. (2007) Do anxiety, body image, social support and coping strategies predict survival in breast cancer? A ten-year follow-up study. *Psychosomatics.*

Ridolfi DR, Crowther JH. (2012) The link between women's body image disturbances and body-focused cancer screening behaviors: A critical review of the literature and a new integrated model for women. *Body Image.*

Lewis-Smith H, Diedrichs PC, Harcourt D. (2018) A pilot study of a body image intervention for breast cancer survivors. *Body Image.*

Bailey KA, Gammage KL, van Ingen C, Ditor D. (2016) Managing the stigma: Exploring body image experiences and self-presentation among people with spinal cord injury. *Health Psychology Open.*

Pinto BM, Trunzo JJ. (2005) Health behaviors during and after a cancer diagnosis. *Cancer.*

De Vries A, Helgeson VS, Schulz T, Almansa J et al. (2019) Benefit finding in renal transplantation and its association with psychological and clinical correlates: A prospective study. *British Journal of Health Psychology*

Adorno G et al. (2018) Positive aspects of having had cancer: A mixed-methods analysis of responses from the American Cancer Society Study of Cancer Survivors-II (SCS-II). *Psycho-oncology*

CHAPTER 9: Pretty healthy

National Eating Disorders Association. Get REAL! About Media and Body Image. A digital media literacy toolkit.

INDEX

✦ ✦ ✦

ACKNOWLEDGEMENTS

✦ ✦ ✦

I love to write and so, for providing me with the opportunity to do so: Jane Morrow, you are my hero. Your guidance and belief in me are priceless. As always, I am so thrilled to be with the entire team at Murdoch Books. To my extraordinary editors Margot Saville and Jane Price, thank you for caring about this book more than I could ever have hoped. And for Carol Warwick and the publicity team, thank you for spreading the word. The cover design by the incredibly talented Alissa Dinallo, with art director Megan Pigott, took my breath away the first time I saw it and does each and every time after that.

My sincere thanks is not enough reward but for Simone Landes and Danica Marcinek at The Lifestyle Suite; your hard work for me never goes unnoticed or unappreciated.

To the many people who have helped me to shape this book and answered my meandering interview questions and clarified the most complex of concepts into priceless pieces of information: outstanding dietitians Rosie Saunt and Helen West from The Rooted Project, Professor Cecilie Thøgersen-Ntoumani (who is also my PhD supervisor and research collaborator/very patient teacher), Alan Flanagan (The Nutritional Advocate), Erin Vogel PhD, Laura Thomas PhD, James Dimmick PhD, Dr Emma Beckett PhD, Professor Ian Caterson, Tyson Tripcony and Peta Adams from Dietitian Life, Professor Diana Harcourt from the Center for Appearance Research, Dr Jasmine Fardouly, Professor Amy Slater and Professor Jennifer Mills and Christina Sabbagh – thank you for sharing your expertise and views with me. I value your time and knowledge immensely and am very grateful to you for sharing your expertise and experiences so openly. To my dear friend, Dr Tara Drummond, who shared her experience of an eating disorder with me so openly: you are a unicorn.

To my many patients over the years, thank you for reminding why I want this world to be a healthier and happier place – to help you.

To all the wonderful people in my life, my friends and family, thank you for your support and love in everything I do. I could not do it without you.